Lose Weight, Feel Great, Look Amazing

Intermittent FASTING

for

Women

OVER *50*

101
Mouthwatering Recipes

and

Useful Tips
To Slim Down Without Dying

KATE RINALDI

TABLE OF CONTENTS

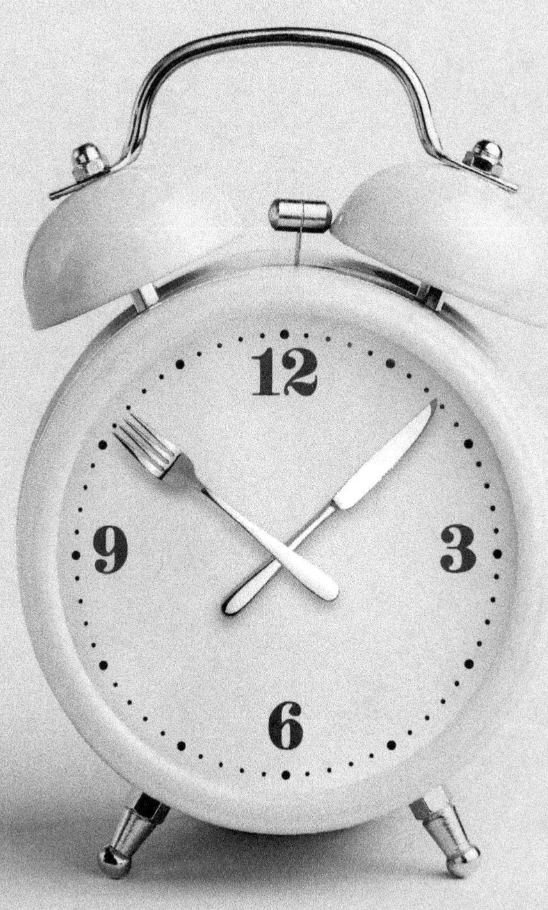

INTRODUCTION

Over the years, intermittent fasting has become more popular, so much that it can now be called a trend of the 21st century. A good factor that made intermittent fasting popular among fitness enthusiasts is that it gives you the freedom and flexibility to eat whatever you want whenever you want to, in as much as it is within your eating window. Over the centuries, the perks offered by this fasting approach has become quite recognized.

Way back since gatherers and hunters' existences, fasting has always been an induced and natural means of survival. In those eras, there were times when it was impossible to find food, forcing the early humans to go for prolonged periods of no meal. Centuries later, this manner of eating has resurfaced and become more popular. In a bid to stay fit and healthy, humans have evolved to adapt to long periods without taking a meal. This has been mainly due to the fact that it has been encouraged to have several health benefits.

Across the globe, there are a lot of people who have attempted to or have gone on intermittent fasting. This could either be as a means of losing and maintaining weight or as a way of fulfilling a religious tenet. However, intermittent fasting is mainly used as a tool for weight control, especially where it concerns losing weight. Therefore, if you are looking to shed some weight and also enjoy the other perks of intermittent fasting, this is the book for you.

Fifty and above are the ages by which women become either peri or post-menopausal. The average for menopause is considered as 52. During this period of menopausal transitioning, the body fat of the woman shifts from the thighs and hips and moves to the lower abdomen. At the same time, women at this age have a lower level of estrogen, which makes their body lose its protection against osteoporosis and heart diseases. The good news now is that intermittent fasting can help women above fifty with fat gain and weight gain as a result of reaching menopause. Intermittent fasting can also help with reducing blood insulin resistance, blood pressure, and blood cholesterol levels. It also helps to improve sleep. Although these have been generally researched, most of the studies that spoken extensively about these benefits were done on women above the ages of fifty.

Written in simple and relatable English, this book will furnish you with information on how to go on intermittent fasting, how it works, why it is right for you, who should do it, and who should not. It is a perfect guide for any beginner seeking to learn and practice intermittent fasting. Let's dive right into it, then.

WHAT IS INTERMITTENT FASTING?

Intermittent fasting is a culture since culture is a way of life. It is simply a manner of living where you fast for a specific period. These periods are usually between meals, but the meals are not as frequent as in our everyday life. When executed correctly, this is a dietary pattern that enables you to lose weight and also allows you several other health benefits. For people who are not interested in losing weight, intermittent fasting helps to maintain their weight while at the same time boosting their energy level.

To put this in context, when on this type of dietary pattern, an individual will stay without food for about 12 to 20 hours, when they can take a meal again. Some people, not beginners, can go for 24 hours without taking anything food just to speed up the process. However, dieters without experience often make the mistake of confusing starvation and fasting. To understand the difference between the two, one has to understand that starvation is an involuntary action. It is the act of depriving your body of food over a long period. This is mostly out of your control. Conversely, fasting is a controlled act of not eating over a specific period that an individual voluntarily go on just for the benefits attached to it.

When it comes to intermittent fasting, the act of staying away from consuming food occurs voluntarily over a period of ten to twelve hours. Another misconception that is very popular is that some people will skip breakfast and call it intermittent fasting. This is a very big misconception that many people have fallen prey to in their bid to convince themselves that they are practicing intermittent fasting. Yes, skipping breakfast can be part of intermittent fasting, but with a special consideration given to the fasting period, eating the right kind of food and not overwhelming the body when you break the fast. Again, when it is rightly executed, there are tonnes of benefits to derive from intermittent fasting.

There exists a very simple logic behind the concept of intermittent fasting. For you to successfully lose weight, your body will need to function on fewer calories. When you choose a specific period for eating, while watching the amount and kind of food that you eat, you are naturally teaching your body to survive on fewer calories. This is because you are consuming less food. The result is that your body becomes calorific deficient. Done with periods of exercise, this act can help you to lose weight considerably. Some of the processes that happen in the body are that your body will undergo hormonal changes that will help it to burn the energy stored as fat.

For people who already have busy schedules around active activities, they can simply incorporate fasting into their daily routine. This is because they are mostly too busy to focus on eating due to their full schedule. This gives them a natural cause to skip a meal or two. The flexibility presented by intermittent fasting, when compared to other dietary plans, motivates and inspires people to choose this fasting approach.

However, as mentioned in the earlier paragraphs, intermittent fasting benefits are not new in the religious world. Religions such as Islam, Judaism, Christianity, Buddhism, and Hinduism all encouraged fasting for one or more days as a spiritual way of becoming more dedicated to God.

However, there is one major disadvantage of intermittent fasting in that you cannot, while practicing intermittent fasting, develop and practice mindful eating. With the self-control improving provision of strict windows for eating, intermittent fasting allows the individuals to eat anything during their feeding window. There are no restrictions to low carbs or fat, neither is there any consideration given to herbs and fruits. The idea is simple, eat less, but eat anything healthy.

Therefore, if your eating period happens to fall in the middle of the night, biting down on a late-night snack stop being a crime, sleeping on a heavy stomach becomes just as accepted. A downside to this is that the body is least active in our state of sleep. Therefore, when you go to bed with a stomach full of heavy and greasy food, you are actually trying to help your body gain weight and not lose it. Sadly, because you have a specific window for eating, you have to eat even if you are not hungry. Fortunately, this is rarely the case.

What happens is that your appetite takes on a pattern, and your body begins to communicate your period of hunger to you. However, you may still experience variations from time to time depending on your hormonal changes, stress level, type and length of exercises, and other environmental factors. Regardless, you can still study your hunger pattern and develop an eating routine that is according to it. In summary, intermittent fasting has several health benefits but may cause you to develop inappropriate eating habits.

Intermittent Fasting: Is it Popular?

In many places all over the world, intermittent fasting has been around for centuries. It is generally considered a practice. But it was not initially regarded or structured as a diet plan. However, experts begin to study it with time. They realized that there are health benefits that such a pattern of eating can provide. As such, they began experimenting with it. It was not until the twenty-first century that the diet became popular, especially in this last decade.

In the year 2012, intermittent fasting gained popularity following the commencement of the TV documentary, 'Eat Fast, Live Longer.' It was a BBC program by Michael Mosley, a journalist with BBC. This was followed by the release of a book called 'The Fast Diet.' Both the show and the book helps shed light on the concept of intermittent fasting, making it gain more popularity across the world. Since then, there have been several other releases on the topic of intermittent fasting that have all helped to booster the popularity of this concept. Some of the most popular include 'The Obesity Code,' released in 2016, and 'The 5'2 Diet' by journalist Kate Harrison in 2013.

As an additional fuel to its already flaming popularity, many prominent figures and celebrities joined the dieting approach. They were successful with it as it helped them to lose weight and stay healthy and fit. With their testimonies, the popularity of intermittent fasting soared. Gradually and slowly, intermittent fasting spread across the globe and soon became a household name. However, most of these were due to the freedom and flexibility that the diet system offered. First, you don't need to watch whether you are eating fat (healthy fat) or carbs. Second, there is no need to count or track calories and macros, and regardless, you will end up losing weight.

It's this freedom and flexibility that makes it a holy grail for people seeking to lose weight. They follow the diet religiously. Across the world, there now exist many online and offline communities of fasters who share experiences and help each other to stay faithful to the ideology that connects them—intermittent fasting. They also help beginners, especially new members, with tips on how to start and stay focused on the diet.

As with many ideologies or practices that concern the health of people, there has been quite a lot of debate on the health risks associated with intermittent fasting. Regardless of its several health benefits and proven weight loss capability, intermittent fasting is still considered as a craze among some factions of the dietary world. Consequently, intermittent fasting has remained a subject of high debate among dietary experts. However, we shall make a brief discussion about the ways that intermittent fasting affects the body based on the available facts.

The main source of energy to the body is carbs stored as sugar. However, in the absence of this, your body began to burn its energy reserve, which at first is stored sugar. Later, when the sugar storage is depleted, the body goes to burning its fat reserves to get energy for the body in the absence of food. This effect of intermittent fasting is so proven and productive that it has passed the test of time and stay around for centuries. There has been real-life evidence of people fasting for long hours and days in a single stretch, and there were not negatively consequential health detriments.

Let's take a look at how intermittent fasting works. When we consume a meal or eat anything, the body absorbs it through the digestion process. It uses some of it for gaining energy for our internal and external activities and excrete the ones that are not needed. The rest of the food is absorbed but not used as sugar, and if in excess, the rest are stored as fat. This is especially when we don't do enough activities, and yet, we eat a lot. The stored energy in either sugar or fat form is used when we do not take food or calories. The storage of energy is done by the hormone known as insulin.

When we eat, the insulin level in the body spikes, which then act to help the body store the energy in the two ways discussed in the last paragraph. Carbs are stored as glucose in the body, and the excesses are stored as fat in the liver and other parts of the body. The extra sugar from carb decomposition is stored as glycogen in the muscles and the liver. The liver does this storage through a process called de-novo lipogenesis, a process through which the liver converts excess glucose into fat for storage in the liver and other parts of the body. Now, there is no limit to how much fat that the body can store. Therefore, as we eat, the body keeps converting the excess sugar into fat storage.

During the period when we refused to eat, the level of insulin in the body drops. This instructs our body to start the process of burning its stored fuels—glucose and fats—for energy. As the body does this, the blood glucose level begins to drop, but the stored energy helps to shore it up back. The body will first use up all the stored glucose in the body. When it is depleted, the body migrates to burning fat deposits. As the body burns these fats, we begin to lose weight. If you fast and simultaneously exercise, the weight loss is faster as the body burns more fat for energy. If you have a busy schedule with active activities as well, the body burns more fats and aids a faster weight loss. Fasting for a longer period also helps.

How Does Intermittent Fasting Affect Hormones and Cells?

Yes, that's what you read. Intermittent fasting can affect you at the cellular and hormonal levels. When you eat, the body releases hormones that help it to coordinate its activities. One such hormone is responsible for the process of burning stored fat for energy. Also, there are general cellular and hormonal changes that place in the body during the period of intermittent fasting. Let's take a look at some of these hormones and what they do.

- The Human Growth Hormone (HGH): During intermittent fasting, the human growth hormone level increases exponentially by a factor of almost five. This increase in the human growth hormone level helps the body to burn fat faster, leading to improved muscle gain.
- Insulin: We already discussed insulin. When the body does not get food, insulin level drops. With this drop, the body's sensitivity to insulin improves. The increased sensitivity helps the body to access and burn stored fat more easily and readily.
- Gene Expression Changes: It is a known fact that cells undergo expressions in their genes that enable them to start repairing damaged parts. When these expressions change, the cells will become more powerful in fighting against diseases. They also become more powerful to support longevity.
- Cellular Repair: During the fasting stages, the activities of the cells towards repairing or removing old protein block from the cells improves. This process is known as autophagy.

How Does Intermittent Fasting Affect Women?

Another hub of several debates, there has been, to date, a constant debate on the topic of intermittent fasting for women. There have been experts who have advised that intermittent fasting as a means of losing weight is bad for women. Yet, there have been other experts who have said that it is safe for women to use intermittent fasting for losing weight.

The truth is that the body undergoes some significant changes in cellular and hormonal levels during intermittent fasting. Now, with hormonal changes, women have the potential to face a number of issues. Some of these issues can manifest in the forms of irregular menstrual cycles, weight gain and weight loss, hair loss, acne, etc.

There have been studies that evidence that insulin and glucose responses in men are more positive compared to the responses in women. This means that intermittent fasting is more effective for weight loss in men than in women. Some sources went as far as to state that intermittent fasting has a caloric restriction that can cause irregular menstrual cycles, reproductive issues, plausible early menopause, and increased stress levels. However, there are no proven researches to back up this claims.

What we know for sure is that there is a major difference in how men react to intermittent fasting as compared to the way that women react to it. It is also established that there is a little risk in women making intermittent fasting an integral part of their overall lifestyle. But all humans are not the same and, as such, respond to intermittent fasting differently. As such, it boils down to the individual responses of people to going on an intermittent fasting routine.

However, health is wealth, and we must pay conscious attention to our bodies. If, as a woman, you intend to go on intermittent fasting, it is important that you do not if you have any of the following conditions;

- Pregnant women should stay off intermittent fasting.
- Women who have never diet or exercise before should not start intermittent fasting first. It is advisable for them to start exercising to see how their body will react first before considering intermittent fasting.
- Women with a history of any form of eating disorders should stay off intermittent fasting.
- Women who have trouble sleeping should avoid going on intermittent fasting.
- Lastly, women who are already suffering from irregular menstrual cycles should also stay away from intermittent fasting.

For women in these categories that are still looking to lose weight, it is advisable to exercise regularly. This will allow you to eat right, burn fat and still lose weight.

Pairing Intermittent Fasting with Keto Diet

Combining intermittent fasting with a keto diet is not unheard of, it is common in individuals who want to lose weight faster than usual. They combine the keto diet with intermittent fasting. The keto diet is a high fat, low carb diet. It works by burning fats into ketones that are used as an energy source by the body, instead of glucose—this act of burning fat results in weight loss. When deprived of carbs, the body fails to produce glycogen and glucose, which fuels the body to produce energy for its various functions. When your body goes into the state of burning fat for ketones, it is said to be in a state of ketosis. When you denied the body of food during intermittent fasting, it goes into a mild state of ketosis. This is an effective way to begin your journey into weight loss.

Intermittent fasting, in some ways, share similarities with going on a keto diet. This is why some people often pair intermittent fasting with the keto diet. How is this done? During the eating period of your intermittent fasting routine, rather than eat foods that are high in carbs as our normal everyday meals, you will substitute them with high-fat, low-carb meals from the keto diet. The carbs in the keto diet are usually between twenty to fifty grams in a day. Eating a keto diet allows you to put your body in ketosis. Fasting helps you sustain ketosis for a long period, thus giving you the ability to burn fat more effectively. What's more? Keto meals are filling, and thus you will feel less hunger.

The Advantages of Intermittent Fasting

1. **Weight Loss**

   As has been discussed, the body uses up its fast deposit as fuel for generating energy when it is not supplied with food. Therefore, if you fast for a longer period, you will burn more fat. Burning more fat means that you will eventually drop some pounds from your body mass. Intermittent fasting, doing just this, remains one of the best means of losing weight. People know that intermittent fasting is powerful when it comes to losing weight and burning fat. This is why most people prefer this approach for losing weight. Another advantage during the weight loss process is that intermittent fasting takes your routine into account and offers you a great degree of flexibility. Reducing the amount of food that you consume means that you are cutting down on calorie intake, making intermittent fasting an effective way of losing weight. There is an additional factor of hormonal level fluctuations that assist in the weight loss process. During intermittent fasting, your body's production of Noradrenaline or norepinephrine increases. Norepinephrine is the hormone that functions to improve your body's fat-burning functionality. As a result, you continuously lose weight as your body burns more fats.

2. **Prolonged Life**

   Intermittent fasting is also famous for enhancing the body's cell longevity and, as a result, prolongs the life of people living this lifestyle. During intermittent fasting, the cells in the body get triggered. When this occurs, the cells function to remove or repair damaged protein blocks, a process that improves the overall wellbeing of the host. Another known fact is that when people go on long periods of calorie restrictions, it helps to lower their risk of developing certain diseases like cancer and hence, helps to boost their overall lifespan.

3. **Reduced Cholesterol and War Against Other Health Issues**

   Another main advantage of intermittent fasting is that it reduces the body's level of cholesterol, amid its other numerous health benefits that help to promote good health. Away from cholesterol, intermittent fasting also reduces the levels of LDL and triglycerides too. And it gets better;

intermittent fasting also prevents some particular chronic issues that post a challenge to good health. It also reduces inflammation. While intermittent fasting is doing all these good works to the body, the level of the person's physical activities is not in any way affected.

4. **No Macronutrient Counting**

When on intermittent fasting, the need to pay attention to what you eat is not there. However, this does not mean that you should not be eating healthy. Unhealthy fat is still not good for your body, and too much of everything still remains detrimental to your health. That said, unlike what is available in some nutrition plans, you don't have any particular limit to the amount of macronutrients that you can include in your meals. As stated earlier in this book, there are restrictions on other diets. For instance, the keto diet is such that if you must lose weight, there is a limit to the amount of carbs that you can take daily, specifically between twenty to fifty grams of carbs. In some other diets, there is a limit to the amount of fatty food that you can consume in order for you to lose weight and improve your health conditions. In all of these other diets, one thing is common; you must adapt to a new way of cooking and eating if you wish to live healthily and lose weight. New ways of cooking and eating mean new recipes and new ingredients in your everyday life if you must stay on these types of diets.

In intermittent fasting, this is not a problem. There is no need for restricting macronutrients when you are on intermittent fasting. You can continue with your eating lifestyle of eating whatever you crave or choose to cook. There are no new recipes or new ingredients. You are free to eat anything that pleases you, in as much as you are eating healthy and safe. It gets better as you can still go on intermittent fasting while you are on a journey. Intermittent fasting does not stop you from frequenting or visiting restaurants, as much as the period you are going to the restaurant to eat falls within your eating window on the intermittent fasting diet plan. Because you can practically eat whatever smells nice and healthy to your nose, you do not have any craving of sort while on an intermittent fasting diet plan.

5. **No Calorie Counting**

Just like as discussed in macronutrients, there is also no need to count calories while on an intermittent fasting diet plan. During a weight loss program on a diet plan, people are often required to regularly count their calorie intake. This is in itself quite a frustrating concept. Some people would have to go as far as using a tracking application and or note to note down all the meals they take. Simultaneously, they will need to maintain a fitness journal in order to track their calorie intake. This happens because of the high tendency of the people on this diet to forget or become too engulfed in their daily lives to have time for counting calories.

With intermittent fasting, the two things you are required to pay attention to and track is your eating period and fasting period. Doing this does not require any special app or consciousness, but rather a formation of a habit of eating at a particular period to which the body becomes adapted and reminds you of it once it is time. Even if the body does not adapt to the periods, it is easier to track than counting calories or macronutrients. And if you are the type that chooses to count calories during intermittent fasting, it is still easier as you can do this in advance, given that you have extended periods between meals. What's more, you do not need to be accurate in your counting. And if you can't do it, it is not compulsory. By its manner of existence, intermittent fasting has automatically restricted your calorie intake by restricting the times you can eat daily to once or twice. Hence, you are already keeping the count of your calories low without even paying any special attention to it.

Disadvantages of Intermittent Fasting

1. **Hunger Pangs**

   It is not rocket science that when you deprived the body of food for a long time, the body will begin to make gurgling sounds. There is also the possibility that you may experience painful pangs of hunger. The good news is that this wave is almost always temporal and will soon pass within an hour or two. The only effort you will need to learn to put in during this phase is controlling the temptation to eat. There is no need for anyone to worry about hunger pangs becoming permanent issues during intermittent fasting as they usually always pass within a short time. Furthermore, as the body begins to adapt to this new style of eating, it also begins to develop a tolerance for hunger when food is not forthcoming. This is why you must give your body time to adapt to such a sudden change in your eating habit. There have been reports from a number of intermittent fasting beginners that the hunger for food increases on the second day to almost an intolerable limit. However, as you keep your resistance up, it begins to recede on the third or fourth day until it eventually vanishes. By the time it has vanished, your body has understood that it needs to start burning the extra fat it has stored up for energy, as food will not be as regular as it used to be anymore. This switch to fat-burning will control your hunger pans and allow you to get through your days without eating.

   It will also help you to increase the amount of your protein in your meals, as doing this will help you to keep the pangs of hunger at bay. It is also advisable that you drink a lot of water during intermittent fasting to avoid doing damages to your kidney as a result of your increased consumption of proteins. It is important to include fiber in your food intake as well, as fibers are known to help keep the stomach filled for longer periods. Fibers also increase your bowel movement, and this helps you to stay away from constipation. Filling up on fibers and proteins gives you the advantage of avoiding hunger pangs in the morning and thus allow you to stay without eating until it is time for lunch.

2. **Constipation**

Constipation is arguably the most common side effect that comes with going on intermittent fasting, especially for those people that keep their eating windows wide apart. When you eat less food, you naturally do not excrete much. Although it may not be a big concern, it is generally advisable that you consult a health practitioner when you feel discomfort in your abdomen, or bloating, or pain. Easing these negative side effects is easy. All you need to do is to use standard laxatives or add magnesium supplements to your diet. There is yet another means of curing constipation. It involves adding more fibrous food to your diet. Such fibrous can include dark vegetables, lentils, bananas, and beans. Again, drinking a lot of water will also help against constipation. Constipation is a quite common side effect at the beginning of switching to an intermittent fasting diet plan. However, once your body becomes used to not getting food at the interval it was hitherto used to, this issue of constipation will eventually go away.

3. **Hypoglycaemia Chances**

Hypoglycemia is a word that described a state of the body where the level of blood sugar is low. It is a typical side effect of intermittent fasting. It is a side effect of skipping meals and eating less food. It is a condition that is often common in individuals that living with diabetes or that are placed on insulin medication. However, hypoglycemia can also happen to people who are neither suffering from diabetes nor placed on insulin medication. When we eat less often, and the level of carbs drop, the amount of sugar available in the body drops drastically as the body is no longer storing sugar. This is why it is important that people who are suffering from diabetes avoid going on intermittent fasting. The presence of hypoglycemia can lead to symptoms like nausea, sweating, dizziness, paleness, uneasiness, and blurred vision. That's not all, it is also not advisable for people with thyroid issues to go on intermittent fasting as they also have a high tendency to suffer from hypoglycemia.

4. **Lean Body Mass Loss (Possible)**

In recent times, debates are beginning to resurface about the possibility of muscle loss alongside fat when people go on intermittent fasting diet plans. For people who are overweight, this is hardly a problem. They merely lose weight by burning fat during the fast stages. However, it is a different ball game for leaner individuals. This set of people will suffer a reduced metabolic rate and a reduction in their lean mass. This is simply because learner people do not have any fat reserve to burn. And with no stored fat to burn, the body targets the muscle mass. The muscle masses are the building block of proteins, which the body can break down into amino acids and use as fuel for generating energy. People who have body fat should not be afraid of this side effect as their muscle mass cannot be targeted by the body. It is only an emergency action by the body and, as such, should not be a major cause for alarm.

5. Stressful

Despite its flexibility and simple approach, intermittent fasting can still be stressful for some people. Some of these people are those who travel frequently and are unable to follow the rules, especially since they will be moving between time zones. Multiple time zone living means that keeping time would not be as easy, and this can result in weight gain, nullifying the reasons for starting intermittent fasting in the first instance.

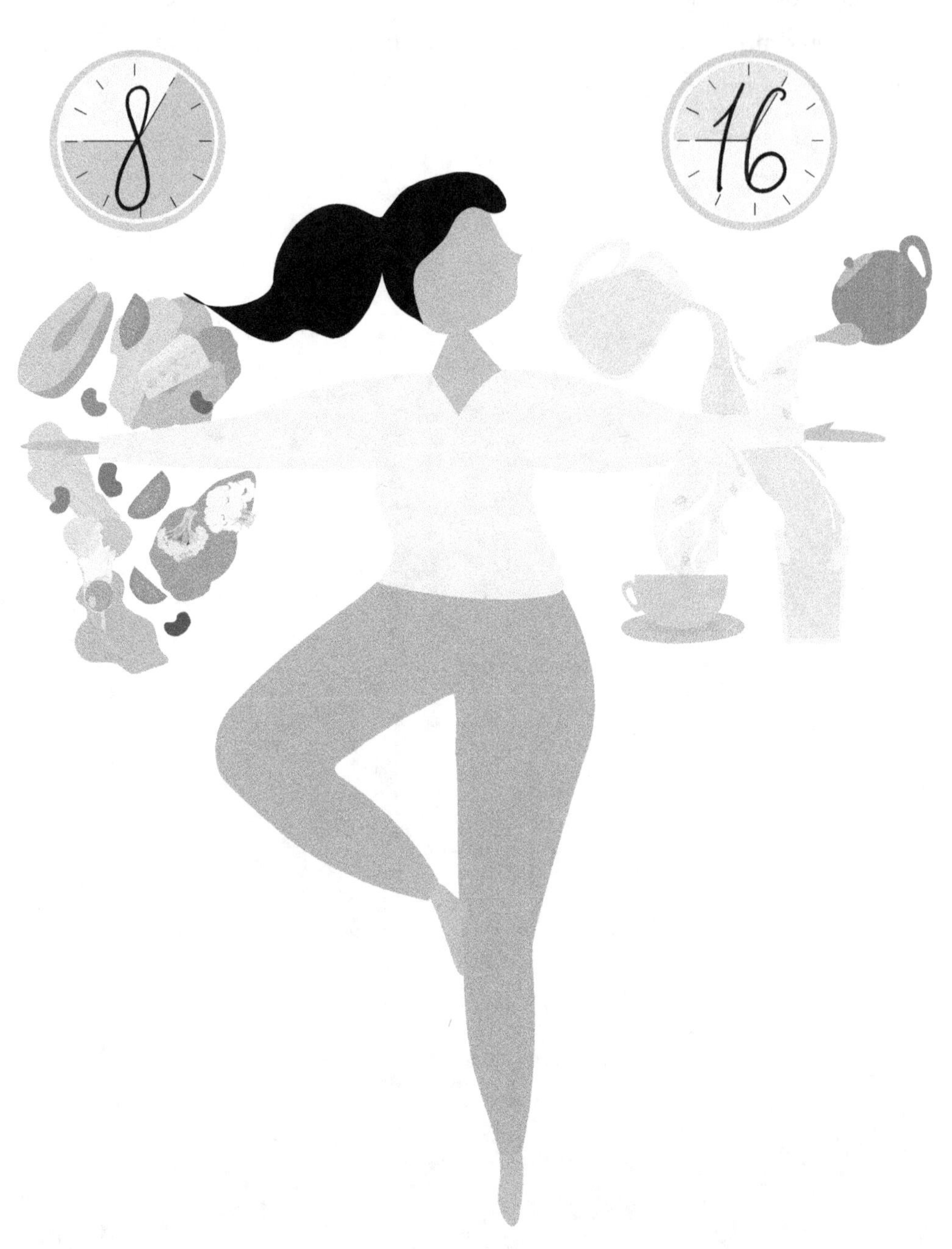

INTERMITTENT FASTING FOR WOMEN OVER FIFTY

For women over the age of fifty, losing weight can be quite a herculean task. This is because women at the ages beyond fifty have a lower metabolism. In addition to this, heavy exercise is not all too advisable as women have achy joints and reduced muscle mass. Some of the women above this age even have sleep issues, if not most of them. However, it is quite beneficial to women at this age to lose fat, especially those dangerous belly fat. Losing belly fat, or any fat at all, can help women over fifty to reduce the risk of serious and dangerous health challenges like heart attacks, cancer, and diabetes.

This is a welcomed advantage. At the ages above fifty, especially for women, the risk of developing a lot of diseases increases. As such, intermittent fasting becomes an advantage. Not only does it minimize the chances of a woman above fifty developing age-related diseases, but it also affords women over fifty a platform above which they can build a fountain of youth through weight loss. In essence, you stay sweet sixteen while also reducing your propensity to develop age-related diseases.

Intermittent fasting is not a scheme to force anyone to go on starving. It does not also mean that you can start consuming any desirable amount of unhealthy food in the periods when you are not fasting. What it does is make you eat within a specified eating window. However, these meals are healthy meals that are steps away from the usual snacks you munch all the time.

For most people practicing intermittent fasting, they schedule their fast in such a way that they spend 12 to 16 hours to fast in a day. In their off-fast period, when they are allowed to eat, they eat normal meals and some intake of periodic snacks. And there is a cherry on top, it does not require too much stress to stick to the eating window; it is not as hard as it sounds. For about eight hours of the fasting period, most of the people practicing intermittent fasting are asleep. During intermittent fasting, especially for women over fifty, it is advisable to drink zero-calorie drinks like coffee, tea, and even water.

Eating Schedule for Women Over Fifty

There are different styles of intermittent fasting that are available to people. These styles are similar, irrespective of age. However, because of the metabolic rate and the fewer muscle mass of women over fifty, I will advise on the plan to work with for efficient weight loss and improved health condition. However, let us quickly discuss the available plans.

The Twelve Hours Intermittent Fasting Plan (12-12)

This intermittent fasting plan involves eating meals that are twelve hours apart. What most people using this plan for intermittent fasting do is to skip breakfast and wait until lunch before they eat again. However, there is no hard and fast rule to this plan or any plan at all. It is all about convenience. There are those on the plan that prefer to have a morning meal. All they do is eat at 7 or 8 am in the morning and wait for 7 or 8 am in the evening to eat again. During this latter style, you must do all you can to avoid late-night snacks as they will fall outside your eating window that starts after 7 or 8, depending on the time you choose between the two. The main idea is to keep your meals twelve hours apart.

The Sixteen Hours Intermittent Fasting Plan (16-8)

This is another intermittent fasting plan. In this plan, the person undergoing intermittent fasting will not eat for sixteen hours. This implies that they have an eating window of eight hours every twenty-four hours. The style that most people on intermittent fasting with this plan adopt is to eat twice in the eight hours' eating window, with a snack or two in between the meals. Choosing your eight hours' eating window is not written in stone either. It is also a matter of convenience. A popular example of this eight hours' eating window is to base the window between noon and eight in the evening. This allows the people using this style to eat a brunch at noon while also taking a late dinner at eight in the evening. Another popular style is the 8-4 eating window style. People on this style stop eating by four in the afternoon and won't taste food until eight the next morning. This sixteen hours intermittent fasting plans helps the dieters to lose weight faster than the twelve hours eating plan.

The Twenty Hours Intermittent Fasting Plan (20-4)

This is definitely not a plan for starters. This intermittent fasting plan involves fasting for a period of twenty hours and having four hours of eating window. Within this four hours of healthy eating, you can eat two or one meal with a snack to feel comfortable. It is almost impossible to eat three meals with this type of fasting plan. It is a plan that is suitable for long-term intermittent fasting individuals, not beginners. Again, there is flexibility with the time, as individuals can base their eating hours on any span of the day. However, it is critical to eat during your peak active hours in order to aid blood insulin level regulation and digestion.

The One-Meal-A-Day Plan (23-1)

The one-meal-a-day plan is also called the twenty-three hours intermittent fasting plan. It involves eating just once a day. This plan does not involve an eating window, as the plan is for the individual to only eat once a day. It does not mean that the individual can eat twice or more during a one-hour eating window. No. What is required is a single meal during a twenty-four hours window, hence why it is not popular as the twenty-three hours intermittent fasting plan.

The 5-2 Schedule for Intermittent Fasting

This is a style that is most helpful to people who are just starting out on intermittent fasting. It involves going on an intermittent fasting plan with rest days. On such rest days, the person is free to eat for as long as they want, but it is advisable to keep the meal healthy. Unhealthy eating on the rest day can do damages to the achievements of the fasting day. The rest day can be a day or two, but two days is the most favored among intermittent fasting enthusiasts. This reason was what birthed the 5-2 schedule for intermittent fasting.

This schedule simply involves the user to go on either the twelve hours intermittent fasting plan or the sixteen hours intermittent fasting plan. However, the users would only abide by this plan for just five days of the available seven days in a week. The other two days are his rest days. The common example is to go on intermittent fasting on the weekdays and then use the weekend days as the rest days. For people who are not always active on weekends, this is not a very good style. It is advisable to fast on a day when you are not mobile or working, as the body does not consume much energy on such days.

Fasting Every Other Day

This is an intermittent fasting plan that involves alternating between days of fasting and days of eating normally. For a person undergoing intermittent fasting using this style, the person can fast on a day and eat on the next day. On the fasting days, it is advisable to keep calories as low as possible. It's quite slow to lose weight using this style, but it does work for weight loss and healthy living. It does not matter the style of fasting that is employed on the fasting day, be it the twelve hours intermittent fasting plan or the fifteen hours intermittent fasting plan. What matters is that the person fasts on one day, using either plan and eat normally on the other days.

Conclusion

For the best result, a person on intermittent fasting needs to be consistent and faithful, as with any other form of diet. However, it is not any harmful to give yourself a break on special occasions. However, if multiple special occasions are occurring consecutively within a short time, it is better to break the fasting for one and stay faithful through the rest. Consistent days of normal eating while on intermittent fasting will damage much of the progress that you have made while on intermittent fasting. This is majorly because your body that has adapted to your new way of eating may have to readjust and adjust again, putting it through unnecessary stress. Also, adjusting and readjusting takes time.

It is best to experiment in order to determine the best plan of intermittent fasting to go on. However, for beginners, the twelve hours intermittent fasting plan and the 5-2 schedule for intermittent fasting are good plans to experiment with. Determining the eating window or time is flexible and can vary from person to person. What individuals should be considerate about is their leisure and business activities. For women above fifty, there is the possibility that most are not working anymore and now stays at home a lot. In order to keep busy, they may have leisure activities in which they invest their time. It thus becomes important that the eating windows fall within their active hours. This ensures that they use the energy up to do these activities, and the spike in the blood level sugar after eating can normalize faster.

Similarly, for those that are still working or have businesses of their own, it is also important that their eating windows fall within their active times. Eating in the active hours does not only help to regulate blood level sugar but it also good for women above fifty as their slow metabolism can be aided by the demand for energy. The overall effect is that they feel good in their body and live a healthier life.

The alternate days fasting plan is also good for beginners, especially for those that are scared of taking the jump. It helps to ease their body into the habit of intermittent fasting. For women above fifty who wish to regulate their body weight as well, the alternate fasting plan is very useful, especially for women above fifty who are not excessively overweight. The sixteen hours intermittent fasting plan is good for people who are already used to the intermittent fasting lifestyle.

Intermittent fasting has another fascinating aspect that most women above fifty can find quite fascinating. This aspect is the ability of intermittent fasting to produce anti-aging effects. The anti-aging effect is achieved through a process primarily known as autophagy. Autophagy is the process through which the body naturally clean out all the damaged cells and replace them with healthy new cells. Wow, you heard right; it is a natural way of cleaning out old cells and replacing them with younger cells. It is like turning back the clock. Autophagy is a part of our being right from time immemorial. The body supplements itself with energy by consuming itself to birth younger cells. Although this cannot last indefinitely, but as you will be eating intermittently, the body does not need to keep it up.

When we go on intermittent fasting, autophagy is increased. The reason for this occurrence is because the cells become stressed during intermittent fasting. This triggers the autophagy process, as it comes in to help in protecting and replenishing the cells.

INTERMITTENT FASTING COOKBOOK

Recipes

Appetizers

Avocado Shrimp Ceviche

Preparation time:
10 MINUTES

Cooking time:
8 MINUTES
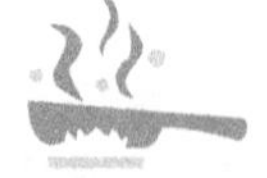

Servings:
4
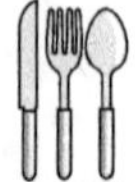

This tasty yet nutritious delicacy is one of the fastest recipes to make in this collection of recommended intermittent fasting dishes. In recent times, people have begun to explore new and unusual possibilities to delight their taste buds, and the avocado shrimp ceviche is a nutritious yet exciting delight for the adventurous and health-conscious eater. The avocado shrimp ceviche combines the tasty delight of shrimp marinated in lime juice with the nutritional advantages of avocados, cilantro, and cucumbers. The avocado shrimp ceviche is an incredible option to start a multiple-course meal with and is quite convenient to make.

Nutritional Information per serving:

Calories 140; Total fat: 7g; Saturated fat: 1.5g; Cholesterol: 115mg; Sodium: 240mg; Carbohydrates: 5g; Fiber: 4g; Sugar: 0g; Protein: 15g.

Ingredients:

- 400 g shelled cooked shrimp
- Two avocados
- Two lemons
- One onion
- One branch of parsley
- Salt
- Pepper

Directions:

1. Cut open the lemons and extract the juices into a bowl.

2. Peel and chop the onion and add the chopped onions to the lemon juice.

3. Marinate the shrimp in lemon juice for 30 minutes. Refrigerate this mixture if possible.

4. Peel and pit the avocados, then dice the flesh. Add the diced avocados to the salad bowl.

5. Chop the parsley and add salt and pepper. Stir the mixture thoroughly

6. Serve the ceviche and enjoy.

Garlic Bruschetta Bread

10 MINUTES 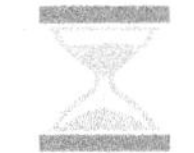

8 MINUTES 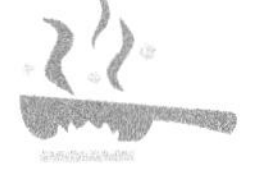

4 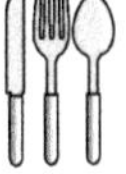

If you are trying to stick to a healthy diet while craving something adventurous, spicy, and fun, then the delicious garlic bruschetta bread is the best choice for you. Made from tomatoes, garlic, and whole-grain bread, this zesty delicacy will definitely leave you craving for more while helping you to keep your calorie levels in check.

Nutritional Information per serving:

Calories 110g; Total fat: 3g; Saturated fat: 0 g; Cholesterol: 0 mg; Sodium: 190mg; Carbohydrates: 18g; Fiber: 1 g; Sugar: 0g; Protein: 3g.

Ingredients:

- Four slices of whole-grain French loaf
- Four tablespoons extra virgin olive oil
- Two cloves garlic
- Four cubed tomatoes
- Eight green or black olives
- Four slices of parmesan cheese
- Eight fresh basil leaves (sliced)
- Thyme
- ½ teaspoon pepper

Directions:

1. Preheat the oven to 350 degrees Fahrenheit.
2. Put the slices of bread in the oven for a few minutes (they should brown a little). Prepare the bread by rubbing a clove of garlic on it. Add a drizzle of olive oil.
3. Cut the fresh tomatoes into cubes and spread the chopped fresh tomatoes on the bread.
4. Add the basil, thyme, olives and pepper, and parmesan cheese
5. Pour in a little olive oil and return to the mix to the oven until the cheese melts.
6. Allow to cook, and enjoy.

Eggplant Dip

45 MINUTES 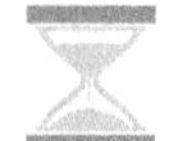

30 MINUTES 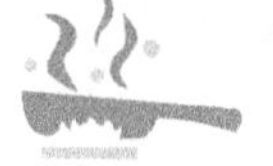

6 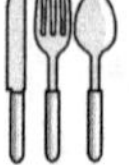

The eggplant is a delicious, nutritious, and easy-to-make appetizer of Middle-eastern origins. Combining the natural goodness of eggplants with the spicy delight of a garlic-based sauce, the eggplant dip is a sure recipe for an unforgettable culinary adventure. The eggplant dip can be enjoyed alone as an appetizer or served alongside pita or crackers as a midday snack.

Nutritional Information per serving:

Calories 77; Total fat: 6g; Saturated fat: 1g; Cholesterol: 0mg;
Sodium: 50mg; Carbohydrates: 6g; Fiber: 3g; Sugar: 2g; Protein:

Ingredients:

- 1 large 1lb eggplant.
- 2 tbsp. extra virgin olive oil
- Two cloves of garlic
- 60 ml (1/4 cup) tahini
- juice of 1 lemon
- ¼ tsp Cayenne pepper
- ¼ tsp. Kosher salt
- 60 ml (1/4 cup) Greek yogurt

Directions:

1. Place the grill at the center of the oven. Preheat the oven to 190 ° C (375 ° F). Line a baking sheet with parchment paper.

2. Slice the top of the garlic head. Brush with olive oil and wrap in foil. Place on the baking sheet.

3. Oil the eggplants and place the flesh side down on the baking sheet. Bake for about 30 minutes with the garlic or until the eggplant flesh is very tender. Let cool.

4. Using a spoon, remove the flesh from the eggplant. In the bowl of a food processor or blender, place the eggplant and press the head of garlic into it to bring out the flesh. Reduce to a puree.

5. Add remaining ingredients.

6. Pepper generously and salt lightly.

Grilled Eggplant with Tomato and Parmesan

Preparation time: 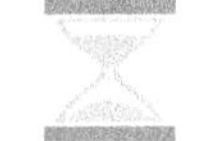

30 MINUTES

Cooking time: 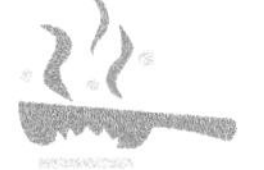

15 MINUTES

Servings: 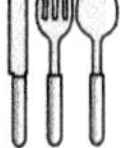

4

This is another appetizer recipe that embodies the tasty nutrition of eggplants and the unbeatable flavors of tomatoes and parmesan cheese. The grilled eggplant with tomato and parmesan has a distinctive taste that will leave you craving for more and is perfect for starting off a multiple-course meal. This smoky snack is perfect for health-conscious individuals as it's low in calories and unhealthy trans-fats.

Nutritional Information per serving:

Calories 237; Total fat: 12g; Saturated fat: 2g; Cholesterol: 7mg; Sodium: 66mg; Carbohydrates: 28g; Fiber: 6g; Sugar: 2g; Protein: 5g.

Ingredients:

- One medium eggplant (sliced into 1-inch slices)
- 1 Box of diced peeled tomatoes
- ½ cup Parmesan cheese
- 5 Fresh basil leaves
- ¼ teaspoons extra virgin olive oil
- ½ tsp. salt.
- ¼ tsp. freshly ground pepper

Directions:

1. Preheat the oven to 410 degrees Fahrenheit (210 ° C). Rinse the eggplants and cut the sliced eggplants lengthwise.

2. Arrange the eggplant slices on the oven rack covered with a sheet of baking paper. Sprinkle them with salt and bake for 10 to 12 minutes.

3. Drain the peeled tomatoes and grate the Parmesan cheese.

4. Rinse and chop the basil.

5. Take the eggplants out of the oven and divide 2 to 3 tbsp of tomatoes. Salt, pepper, sprinkle with parmesan, and toast in the oven for 3 to 4 min.

6. Drizzle with olive oil, sprinkle generously with chopped basil, and serve immediately.

Salads, Soups, And Sandwiches

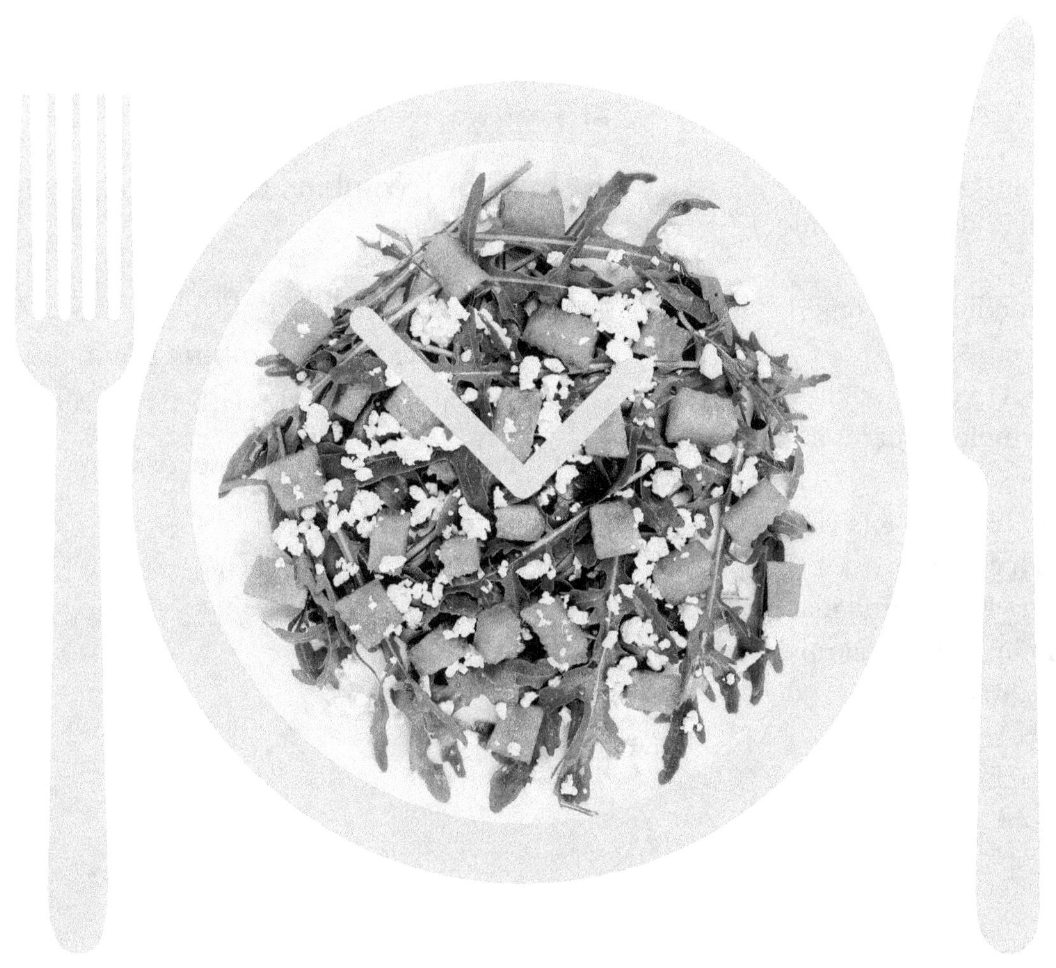

Watermelon and Feta Salad

Preparation time: 10 MINUTES 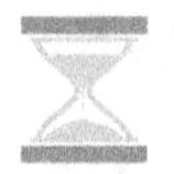 | **Cooking time:** 0 MINUTES 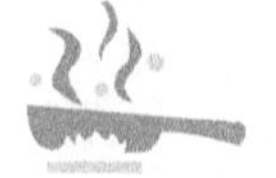 | **Servings:** 4 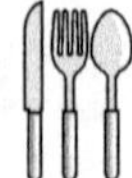

This simple and refreshing dish combines the natural fruity goodness of watermelons and a distinctive blend of cheese, olive oil, and onions. The watermelon feta salad is perfect as a healthy early morning starter dish or as a relaxing evening delight. The watermelon and feta salad helps you stay sufficiently hydrated and is filled with beneficial plant compounds that improve cardiac health and reduce your susceptibility to cancers.

Nutritional Information per serving:

Calories 128; Total fat: 4g; Saturated fat: 2g; Cholesterol: 13mg; Sodium: 222mg; Carbohydrates: 16g; Fiber: 2g; Sugar: 0g; Protein: 6g.

Ingredients:

- 1/3 cup (75 ml) olive oil
- 30 ml (2 tbsp.) Balsamic vinegar
- 1/2 medium red onion (minced)
- 750 ml (3 cups) seedless watermelon, cut into 1-inch cubes
- 1 cup (250 ml) feta cheese in 1-inch cubes
- 1 liter (4 cups) arugula
- 1/4 cup (60 ml) pumpkin seeds (toasted)
- ½ tsp. sea salt
- ½ tsp. freshly ground pepper

Directions:

1. In a bowl, combine the olive oil, vinegar, and onion.
2. Add in the salt and pepper.
3. In a serving plate, combine the melon, feta, and arugula. Drizzle with vinaigrette.
4. Garnish with pumpkin seeds.

Filet mignon Salad

Preparation time: 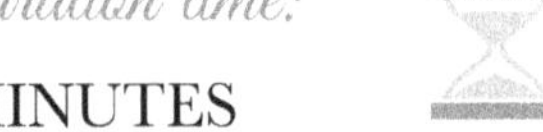
20 MINUTES

Cooking time: 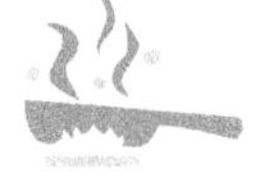
15 MINUTES

Servings: 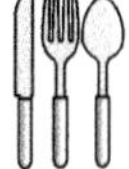
1

Oh, the filet mignon!!! We all know it; we have all tasted it or planned to eat it at a point in the not so distance future. We have added greens and goat cheese, and tomatoes to transform it into a salad. Never thought of that, right? Wait till you taste it.

Nutritional Information per serving:

Total Carbs: 12.7g; Protein: 36.6g; Fat: 77.1g; Fibre: 4.1g; Sodium: 602mg; Calories: 910

Ingredients:

- ¼ cup of fresh chopped basil
- ¼ chopped large head of romaine lettuce
- ½ cup of rice wine vinegar
- ½ trimmed and thinly sliced (crosswise) large head Belgian endive
- ½ pound of filet mignon
- ½ tbsp. of sea salt
- 1 ½ tbsp. of olive oil
- 1 ½ cups of baby arugula
- 1 tbsp. of grass-fed butter, unsalted
- 2 ounces of crumbled goat cheese
- 2 tbsp. of pure maple syrup
- 8 halved cherry tomatoes

Directions:

1. Mix the basil, endive, arugula, and romaine in a large salad bowl and set aside.

2. Pour the maple syrup, rice wine vinegar, pepper, salt, and lemon juice into a food processor. Run it at slow speed while adding in about ½ cup of the olive oil. Take it out of the processor and set it aside.

3. In a cast iron skillet on medium heat, melt the butter with the left-over olive oil for a minute. Then add the filet mignon and cook each side for 7 minutes to your desired level of "done."

4. Take it off the skillet and let it cool for 5 minutes before slicing into strips.

5. Add the tomatoes, filet mignon, and goat cheese into a salad bowl. Pour in the mix from the other salad bowl and toss well to ensure everything is sufficiently coated. Serve.

Asian Strawberry Salad

15 MINUTES

Cooking time:
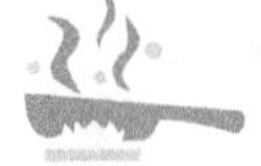

0 MINUTES

Servings:

4

The Asian strawberry salad is a healthy exotic delicacy that combines the delightful taste of strawberries with the nutritional power of Spinach. This recipe is pretty easy to make from easy-to-find nutrients. This dish is also loaded with antioxidants, vitamins, and essential minerals, making it a perfect dietary choice for individuals of all ages.

Nutritional Information per serving:

Calories 580; Total fat: 36g; Saturated fat: 6g; Cholesterol: 0 mg; Sodium: 280mg; Carbohydrates: 45g; Fiber: 6g; Sugar: 23g; Protein: 26g

Ingredients:

- 160 g baby spinach or baby spinach or four handfuls
- 160 g of bean sprouts
- 100 g strawberries or 20 small strawberries
- 40 g unsalted peanuts

Asian Dressing Sauce:

- 2 tbsp. sesame oil
- 1 tbsp. tablespoon or tablespoon of soy sauce reduced in salt
- 1 tbsp. rice vinegar
- 1 tbsp. lemon juice
- 1 tbsp. coffee or teaspoon of liquid honey
- 1/4 teaspoon. grated kaffir lime or teaspoon

Directions:

1. In a small bowl, mix the honey with the rice vinegar and lemon juice, add the soy sauce and sesame oil.

2. Grate the kaffir lime in a small container and add the zest to the sauce.

3. Wash and wring out the spinach leaves.

4. Wash and drain the bean sprouts.

5. Wash and hull the strawberries, then cut them into halves.

6. Place the spinach leaves and bean sprouts in a bowl. Add the vinaigrette sauce, mix. Add the strawberries and peanuts, mix gently. You can also divide your seasoned salad between bowls and then sprinkle the strawberries and peanuts before serving.

Vegan Chili

<table>
<tr>
<td>Preparation time:
1 HOUR</td>
<td>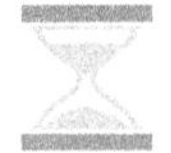</td>
<td>Cooking time:
50 MINUTES</td>
<td>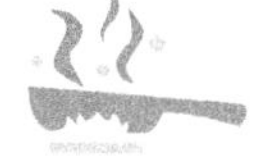</td>
<td>Servings:
2</td>
<td>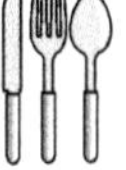</td>
</tr>
</table>

This is a plain good old chili soup with a lot of vegetables. For extra protein, you may choose to include ground turkey or beef in the recipe. You would, however, have to cook the beef with the onions from the beginning.

Nutritional Information per serving:

Total Carbs: 41.0g; Protein: 10.7g; Fat: 7.5g; Fibre: 12.6g; Sodium: 1,188mg; Calories:263

Ingredients:

- ¼ cup of olive oil
- 1 cup of tomato juice
- 1 cup of peeled carrots
- 1 tbsp. of ground ancho chili pepper
- 1 chopped chipotle in adobo
- 1 tbsp. of chopped garlic
- 1 can of roughly chopped plum tomatoes
- 2 tbsp. of fresh chopped cilantro
- 2 chopped medium-sized jalapenos
- 2 tbsp. of salt
- 2 tbsp. of red onions, finely chopped
- 2 cups of chopped assorted bell peppers, seeded
- 2 cups of chopped yellow onion
- 1 can of rinsed and drained red kidney beans
- 1 can of rinsed and drained black beans
- 1 can of rinsed and drained cannellini beans
- 4 tbsp. of ground cumin

Directions:

1. Heat the olive oil in a large, heavy-bottomed Dutch oven over medium heat. Pour in the chopped carrot, diced onions, and bell peppers. Season with salt and cook for 15 minutes on medium heat till the onions become translucent.

2. Get a small skillet going on medium heat. Toast the cumin in the skillet for about 1 minute, then transfer it into the pot with the onions and carrots.

3. Add the chipotle, ancho, garlic, and jalapenos to the pot as well and cook for 5 more minutes.

4. Pour in the beans, tomato juice, and tomato and stir. Reduce to low heat and allow everything to simmer for 45 minutes.

5. Garnish with cilantro and red onions when serving.

Lemon and Ginger Juice with Fruit Salad

10 MINUTES 

0 MINUTES 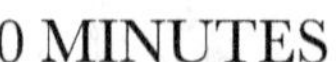

2 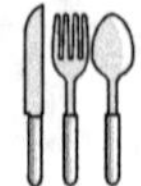

Everyone knows how a regular fruit salad looks like, and this is a fruit salad with a difference. We are going to add a different dimension to how it tastes. Think fruit salad with the spicy ginger taste and sour, the tangy feel of the lemon juice. This would raise your salad experience to a whole new height.

Nutritional Information per serving:

Total Carbs: 74.1g; Protein: 5.0g; Fat: 17.9g; Fibre: 14.3g; Sodium: 46mg; Calories:459

Ingredients:

- ¼ cup of raw cacao nibs
- ½ cup of unsweetened shredded coconut
- 1 cup of pineapple chunks
- 1 cup of seeded and peeled cantaloupe
- 1 cup of sliced green seedless grapes
- 1 medium-sized peeled and sectioned grapefruit
- 1 medium-sized chopped Granny Smith apple
- 1 cup of peeled and cubed honeydew melon
- 2 tbsp. of freshly grated ginger
- 3 tbsp. of freshly squeezed lemon juice

Directions:

1. Get a large bowl and mix all the ingredients together.
2. Toss and mix thoroughly.
3. Divide the mix into two salad bowls and serve.

Fried Tofu and Tuna Salad

Preparation time: 25 MINUTES 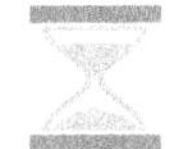 | **Cooking time:** 15 MINUTES 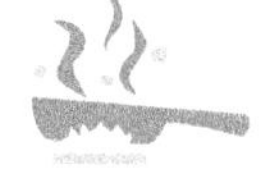 | **Servings:** 4 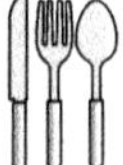

This simple yet delicious delicacy is a perfect addition to an intermittent fasting diet. This simple salad combines the nutritional powers of Tofu with the distinctive taste of tuna to give a truly wholesome and flavorful salad. Tuna is an exceptional source of Vitamin D, with a mere three ounces of tuna giving more than half of the required daily intake of this essential vitamin. Tuna is also highly loaded with iron, which improves blood health, and iodine, which helps prevent goiter. Tofu, on the other hand, is packed with essential minerals, including manganese, copper, and zinc.

Nutritional Information per serving:

Calories 461; Total fat: 17g; Saturated fat: 1g; Cholesterol: 51 mg; Sodium: 779mg; Carbohydrates: 15g; Fiber: 2g; Sugar: 7g; Protein: 60g.

Ingredients:

- One packet of Tofu
- 2 tbsp. flour
- One egg white
- 2 tbsp. breadcrumbs
- One curly salad
- ½ cucumber
- Two tomatoes
- One can of tuna
- 1 tbsp. balsamic vinegar
- 4 tbsp. extra virgin olive oil
- 5 tbsp. regular frying oil

Directions:

1. Cut the Tofu into 1 cm slices and coat them in the flour, then in the egg white, and then in the breadcrumbs.

2. Fry the tofu slices in regular frying oil at 180° C until they become golden brown.

3. Cut the cucumber and tomatoes into thin slices and add them to the fried Tofu.

4. Add the tuna and mix. Mix the balsamic vinegar with the olive oil.

5. Arrange everything on the plates and finish with the balsamic vinegar dressing.

Sweet Potatoes and Mustard Greens with Smoky Black-Eyed Pea Soup

Preparation time: 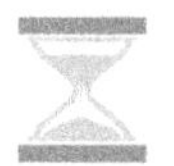
2 H 45 MINUTES

Cooking time: 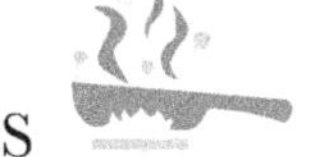
2 H 30 MINUTES

Servings: 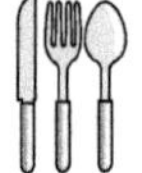
2

The soup offers a lot of flexibility in your choice of ingredients. If you so desire, you can switch the collard greens with Julienned Kale or even the frozen mustard greens with dark fresh leafy greens if that is your preference. Whichever path you choose to take with this soup, you are still going to get the delicious savory taste of the peas and the soothing earthiness of the greens.

Nutritional Information per serving:

Total Carbs: 18.6g; Protein: 4.8g; Fat: 2.4g; Fibre: 5.2g; Sodium: 1,283mg; Calories:107

Ingredients:

- ¼ tbsp. of fresh chopped cilantro
- 1 large size chopped carrot
- 1 dried chipotle chili
- 1 large, sweet 4potato
- 1 tbsp. of olive oil
- 1 tbsp. of dried thyme
- 1 pound of washed dried black-eyed peas
- 1 package of chopped frozen mustard greens.
- 1 can of drained diced tomatoes
- 1 medium sized chopped yellow onion
- 1 tbsp. of ground cumin
- 2 bay leaves
- 2 tbsp. of salt
- Chopped 2 medium sized celery stalk
- 2 quarts of vegetable stock
- 2 tbsp. of dried oregano

Directions:

1. Carefully wash and peel the potatoes. Then cut them into 1-inch cubes. Set them aside.

2. Heat the olive oil in a large, heavy bottomed Dutch oven over medium heat. Pour in the chopped carrot, diced onions, and celery. Season with salt and cook for 5 minutes. When the onions become translucent, add the cumin, dried oregano, bay leaves, chipotle chili, and thyme, then cook for 2 more minutes.

3. Pour in the vegetable stock and the black-eyed pea into the mix. Increase the heat to high. Once it boils over, reduce the heat to low and allow it to simmer for 2 hours till the peas become very soft.

4. Add the potato cubes and cook for an additional 20 minutes. Then introduce the tomatoes and chopped mustard greens and cook till the mustard greens and potatoes are tender. You can adjust the consistency of the broth by adding more vegetable stock. The stock should ideally have a lot of broth.

5. Once the broth is done, remove the bay leaves. Garnish with the chopped cilantro and serve.

Couscous Salad With Black Beans

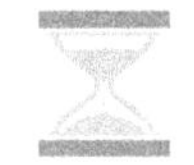 **Preparation time:**
25 MINUTES

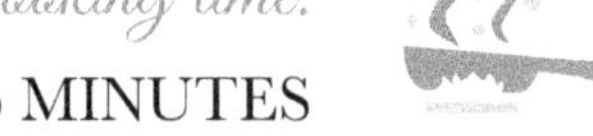 **Cooking time:**
15 MINUTES

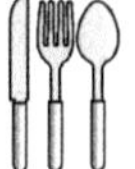 **Servings:**
8

Black beans, a special component of this recipe, is especially rich in folate, potassium, and Vitamin B6, making it a nutritionally packed meal option. Couscous, on the other hand, is rich in selenium, making it useful in the retardation of the activities of free radicals in the body while also preventing the risks of cancers and cardiac diseases. Couscous salad and black beans have also been proven to improve the body's immunity and general resistance to disease. This simple dish is easy to prepare, has a great unbeatable taste, and can be kept conveniently in a refrigerator for up to four days.

Nutritional Information per serving:

Calories 490; Total fat: 6g; Saturated fat: 1 g; Cholesterol: 0 mg;
Sodium: 880 mg; Carbohydrates: 87g; Fiber: 1g; Sugar: 11g; Protein: 24g.

Ingredients:

- 1 1/4 cup chicken broth
- 1 cup raw couscous
- 3 tbsp. tablespoons extra virgin olive oil
- 2 tbsp. lime juice
- 1 cup red wine vinegar
- 1/2 tsp. cumin powder
- Eight green onions, chopped
- One red pepper, seeded and cut into small pieces
- 1/4 cup chopped cilantro
- 1 cup of thawed corn
- 400g canned black beans, drained
- ½ tsp. Salt
- ¼ tsp. freshly ground pepper

Directions:

1. In a saucepan, bring the chicken broth to a boil and stir in the couscous. Cover and remove from heat. Let sit for 5 minutes.

2. In a large bowl, combine the olive oil, lime juice, vinegar, and cumin. Add the green onions, red pepper, cilantro, corn, and beans; stir well.

3. Separate the couscous seeds with a fork. Add to the other ingredients in the bowl and stir again.

4. Season, taste, and serve (or refrigerate).

Citrus Bulgur Salad

Preparation time: 
2 H 15 MINUTES

Cooking time: 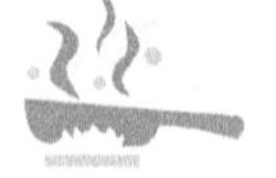
15 MINUTES

Servings: 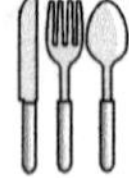
4

The easy-to-prepare citrus bulgur salad combines the low-calorie and high-fiber content of bulgur wheat with the zesty flavor of orange, line, and grapefruit to give a tasty and nutritious salad for all seasons. The citrus bulgur salad is loaded with sodium for optimal functioning of the central nervous system and for maintaining a healthy balance of water and minerals in the body. The salad also features a healthy amount of fiber, promoting a healthy gut and rapid digestion. The salad contains basically zero cholesterol and low levels of saturated fats, making it an exceptionally healthy option for the entire family.

Nutritional Information per serving:

Calories 380; Total fat: 18g; Saturated fat: 2g; Cholesterol: 0mg;
Sodium: 230mg; Carbohydrates: 47g; Fiber: 12g; Sugar: 8g; Protein: 12g.

Ingredients:

- 250g bulgur
- 250g cherry tomatoes
- One bell pepper
- One bunch of spring onions
- One handful of broad beans (fresh shelled)
- One bunch of mint
- One can of tuna in brine
- Two limes
- One orange (small)
- One grapefruit (small)
- 1 tbsp. turmeric
- Ten drops of Tabasco
- 5 tbsp. of olive oil
- ¼ tsp. Salt
- ¼ tsp. freshly ground black pepper

Directions:

1. Cook the bulgur for 10 minutes in a pot of salted boiling water with one tablespoon of turmeric. Drain in a colander, let cool.
2. Wash, dry, chop the mint (keep a few sprigs for decoration).
3. Take the zest of the limes, cut it into thin sticks. Squeeze the lemons, grapefruit, and orange.
4. Wipe and dice the pepper after removing the seeds and white parts.
5. Wash, dry the tomatoes, divide them in 2.
6. Clean the spring onions by removing the first leaves and keeping part of the tail. Cut them into slices.
7. Pour the bulgur into a salad bowl, add ten drops of Tabasco, lemon zest, and citrus juice. Mix.
8. Add tomatoes, peppers, beans, and onion. Mix thoroughly.
9. Add the drained tuna, chopped mint, salt, and pepper. Stir thoroughly.
10. Drizzle with olive oil, mix well again, cover, refrigerate for 2 hours.
11. Serve the bulgur salad in glasses, garnish with a sprig of mint.

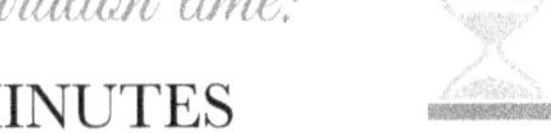

Preparation time:

10 MINUTES

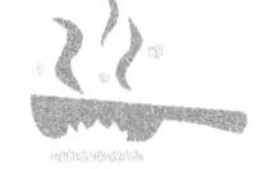

Cooking time:

6 MINUTES

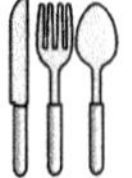

Servings:

2 ½ CUPS

The curry dips are an awesome replacement for your regular dips. If you love hot spicy dips, you can add jalapenos to the ingredients. You can use green peppers instead if you are not one for spicy dips.

Nutritional Information per Half Cup:

Total Carbs: 4.2g; Protein: 0.7g; Fat: 17.2g; Fibre: 0.8g; Sodium: 257mg; Calories:174

Ingredients:

- 1/8 tbsp. of freshly squeezed lemon juice
- 1/8 tbsp. of cayenne pepper
- ¼ tbsp. of salt
- ½ tbsp. of ground turmeric
- ½ cup of finely diced yellow onion
- ½ tbsp. of ground coriander
- ½ medium sized diced jalapeno that has been seeded and stemmed
- 1 tbsp. of olive oil
- 1 tbsp. of ground cumin
- 1 tbsp. of fresh chopped cilantro
- 1 tbsp. of curry powder
- 1 tbsp. of water
- 1 tbsp. of raisins, soft
- 1 ½ cups of mayonnaise
- 2 tbsp. of diced seeded red bell pepper

Directions:

1. With the burner set on medium heat, place a skillet over the burner and heat the olive oil for 30 seconds before adding the red bell pepper, onion, and jalapeno. Stir constantly for 5 minutes till the onions become translucent.

2. Add the coriander, turmeric, cumin, cayenne pepper, curry powder, and salt and cook for a minute till the aroma of the spices become evident. Add water and the raisins, then mix.

3. Pour everything into a food processor and pulse on high speed for 30 seconds. Scrape down the sides of the food processor till all the mixture stuck on the sides are at the bottom of the bowl. Add the cilantro and mayonnaise and process again for 30 secs till it has an even and smooth consistency.

4. Add the lemon juice to the mixture and serve.

Split Pea Soup

3 H 30 MINUTES

 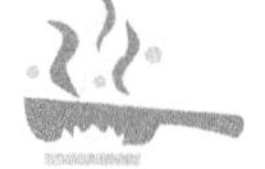

15 MINUTES

 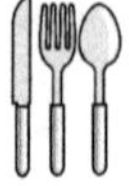

4

Peas are a fantastic source of antioxidants that help to reduce the oxidative effects of unhealthy free radicals in the body. Therefore, peas can help to reduce the effects of aging and greatly strengthen body immunity. Peas are also rich sources of Vitamins C and E, which help in the healing of wounds and in boosting fertility, and in the reduction of oxidative damage. Split pea soup is a delicious intermittent fasting dish that is pretty easy to put together. With an actual preparation time of just 20 minutes and an easy-to-follow recipe, you simply can't go wrong with the split pea soup.

Nutritional Information per serving:

Calories 230; Total fat: 2.5g; Saturated fat: 0 g; Cholesterol: 0 mg; Sodium: 660 mg; Carbohydrates: 38g; Fiber: 13g; Sugar: 8g; Protein: 14g.

Ingredients:

- 200g split peas
- Two carrots
- Three onions
- One clove of garlic
- One stalk of celery
- One bunch of parsley
- One bay leaf
- 25 cl milk or liquid cream
- 5 tbsp. cooking oil

Directions:

1. Wash the split peas and soak in hot water for 1 hour.

2. Drain the peas and put them in a saucepan filled with 1 liter of water. Bring the peas to boil, set the cooker on low heat, and then cook for 2 hours. Add salt 1 hour into the cooking process.

3. In the meantime, grate the carrots, chop the onions and parsley, slice the garlic clove, and cut the celery into small cubes. Add this mixture to the cooked peas.

4. Heat the cooking oil in a sauté pan and heat the vegetables for 10 minutes until they are brown. Add the vegetables to the pea soup, then add in pepper and the bay leaf. Let the mixture sit for 5 minutes.

5. Put the entire mixture in a soup blender, add the milk or cream and serve immediately.

Tuscan White Bean Soup

Preparation time: 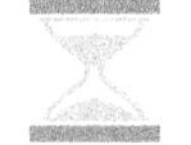
1 H 30 MINUTES

Cooking time: 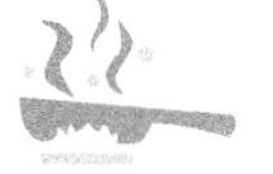
1 H 15 MINUTES

Servings: 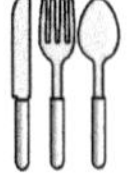
2

The sumptuous broth would have you feeling full and satisfied for a long time. The fibers in the beans help keep hunger away while providing the much-needed protein for a healthy body.

Nutritional Information per serving:

Total Carbs: 36.3g; Protein: 15.4g; Fat: 5.1g; Fibre: 8.2g; Sodium: 1,379mg; Calories:237

Ingredients:

- ¼ tbsp. of salt
- ¼ tbsp. of ground white pepper
- 1 bay leaf
- 1 diced medium sized yellow onion
- 1 large shredded leek (only the white parts)
- 2 cups of large white beans that have been soaked overnight
- 2 tbsp. of olive oil
- 3 shredded cloves of garlic
- 3 quarts of vegetable stock
- 3 tbsp. of chopped fresh rosemary

Directions:

1. With the burner on medium heat, place a large soup pot on it and add 1 tablespoon of olive oil. Heat the oil for one minute, then add the garlic, onions, and leek. Stir frequently while cooking for approximately 10 minutes till the onions become translucent. Add the bay leaf and the rosemary to the pot and continue cooking for five more minutes.

2. Pour in the vegetable stock and the soaked white beans into the pot and boil at high heat. Once the stock boils, bring the heat to low and cook the broth for an hour till the beans become very soft and marshy.

3. Take the pot off the burner and remove the bay leaf from the broth. Divide the soup into three parts. Pour two parts in the blender and puree. Add the puree back to the remaining soup and season with salt and pepper.

4. Sprinkle one tablespoon of olive oil equally on the bowls of soup when serving.

Lentil Soup

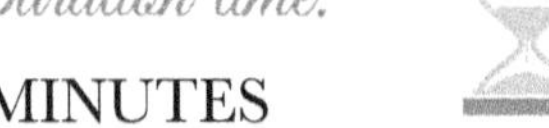

20 MINUTES

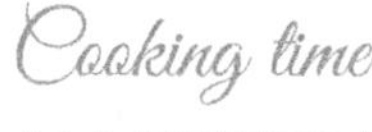
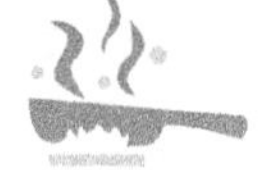

15 MINUTES

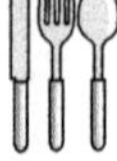

1

Lentil soup is a nutritious and tasty delicacy that fits perfectly into the goals of the intermittent fasting diet. Lentil soup is an intermittent fasting recipe that can be cooked quite rapidly; this soup takes just fifteen minutes. Lentil soup is also packed with a bunch of important nutrients, including B Vitamins and zinc. The magnesium in the lentil soup boosts bone health and promotes healthy teeth. The potassium improves nervous system functioning, and the zinc helps in boosting immunity and reducing susceptibility to disease. Lentil soup is also a fantastic source of plant-based proteins, which are lacking in most modern foods consumed in most contemporary societies. Lentil soup is also rich in fiber, aiding digestion and rapid absorption of food nutrients.

Nutritional Information per serving:

Calories 230; Total fat: 3.5 g; Saturated fat: 0 g; Cholesterol: 0 mg; Sodium: 350 mg; Carbohydrates: 39 g; Fiber: 7g; Sugar: 8 g; Protein: 13g.

Ingredients:

- Two onions, finely chopped
- Two garlic cloves, finely chopped
- ½ tsp. curry powder
- 1 tbsp. Extra virgin olive oil
- Two carrots, peeled and cut.
- 5 cups chicken broth
- 3/4 cup red lentils (rinsed)
- ¼ tsp. ground pepper

Directions:

1. Heat the olive oil in a saucepan over medium-high heat.
2. Gently fry the onions in the hot oil until they are slightly browned, then add in garlic and curry.
3. Add the carrots and cook for 1 minute, stirring constantly. Add the remaining ingredients.
4. Boil the entire mixture, cover, and let simmer gently for 10 minutes.
5. Add seasonings sparingly, and enjoy with pitas.

Falafel Sandwich with Lentils and Avocado Sauce

Preparation time: 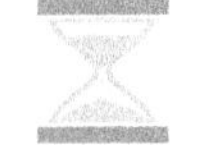
1 H 20 MINUTES

Cooking time: 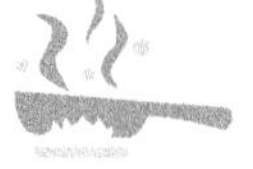
50 MINUTES

Servings: 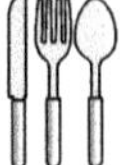
10

This special falafel sandwich dish combines the tasty goodness of falafels with the nutritional powers of lentils and avocados. The falafel sandwich has minimal calories and trans fats and has a healthy dose of proteins for tissue building, fibers for easy digestion and preventing constipation, magnesium for promoting strong bones and teeth, and zinc for reducing susceptibility to disease.

The falafel sandwich with avocado sauce is not only highly nutritious, but it is also a refreshing snack that is easy to put together, with a total cooking time of only 40 minutes.

Nutritional Information per serving:

Calories 428; Total fat: 21g; Saturated fat: 2g; Cholesterol: 1mg; Sodium: 607mg; Carbohydrates: 50g; Fiber: 8g; Sugar: 7g; Protein: 14g.

Ingredients:

- ¾ cup of brown lentils
- 1 cup tahini
- 1 cup tightly packed fresh cilantro leaves
- 1 cup firmly packed flat-leaf parsley
- 2 tbsp. tablespoon olive oil
- One clove of garlic
- ¼ cup lemon juice
- 1 tsp. sea salt
- 1 to 2 tsp. flour (gluten-free, if needed)

Green avocado sauce
- One ripe avocado
- ¼ cup organic non-roasted cashews (soaked in lukewarm water for 30 minutes)
- ½ cup mixed parsley and cilantro
- One clove of garlic
- ½ cup of water
- ½ cup olive oil
- ¼ tsp. Freshly ground pepper, to taste

Directions:

1. After rinsing the lentils, put them in a saucepan and add enough water to cover the lentils.

2. Bring the lentils to a boil, then simmer over low heat for 20 to 30 minutes. It is critical for the lentils to remain submerged in the water throughout cooking.

3. Preheat the oven to 190 ° C (375 ° F).

4. Once the lentils are cooked, mix all the ingredients in a food processor, except the flour. The preparation should be still grainy and with pieces of lentils, but it should be possible to form balls easily.

5. Stir in the flour, one teaspoon at a time, then form 10 balls.

6. On a baking sheet covered with parchment paper, place the falafels and bake for 20-25 minutes. You can also heat them in hot oil for 5 to 7 minutes in a non-stick pan.

7. Serve the falafels with avocado sauce as a dip or as a sandwich on naan or pita bread, topped with Boston lettuce, grated carrots, sprouts, and sauce, if desired.

Portobello Mushroom Burgers

Preparation time: 
30 MINUTES

Cooking time: 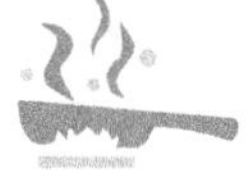
8 MINUTES

Servings: 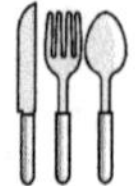
4

If you are trying to keep the calories low while sticking mainly to vegetables, but you still want a burst of adventure at the same time, then Portobello mushroom burgers are definitely the way to go. These handy, healthy snacks contain moderate amounts of fat, no cholesterol, and healthy amounts of protein for bodybuilding, and healthy carbohydrates for energy. The nutritional composition of Portobello mushroom burgers makes them great for adventurous eaters trying to lower their risk of heart disease and obesity while building immunity against diseases. Portobello mushroom burgers are not only packed with essential nutrients, but they also taste amazing, combining the distinctive flavor of mozzarella with the satisfying taste of mushrooms. This snack requires only thirty-five minutes of total cooking time.

Nutritional Information per serving:

Calories 330; Total fat: 17g; Saturated fat: 2.5g; Cholesterol: 0mg; Sodium: 650mg; Carbohydrates: 41g; Fiber: 3g; Sugar: 7g; Protein: 11g.

Ingredients:

- ¼ cup balsamic vinegar
- 2 tbsp. tablespoon olive oil
- ½ tsp. Dried basil
- ½ tsp. dried oregano
- One cup chopped garlic
- ½ tsp. Salt
- ¼ tsp. ground pepper
- Four Portobello mushroom caps
- Four slices of Mozzarella or Provolone cheese

Directions:

1. In a shallow container, whisk together vinegar, oil, basil, oregano, garlic, salt, and pepper.
2. Place the mushrooms in the preparation, soaking them well. Let sit at room temperature for about 15 minutes, turning the mushrooms twice.
3. Preheat barbecue to medium-high heat.
4. Place the mushrooms on the barbecue, reserving the marinade. Cook, 5 to 8 minutes per side, until the mushrooms are tender. Brush frequently with marinade.
5. Two minutes before the end of cooking, garnish with cheese.
6. At the same time, put the bread on the grill to lightly brown it.
7. Remove from heat and garnish with condiments (mayonnaise, ketchup, mustard).
8. Insert a toasted mushroom in each bun and garnish with tomatoes, salad and onions. (optional).

Artichoke dip

Preparation time: 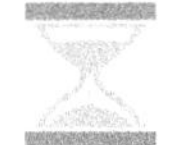	Cooking time: 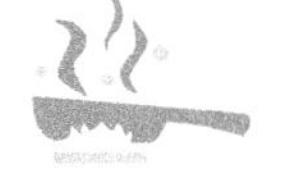	Servings: 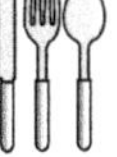
55 MINUTES	45 MINUTES	1

This is very much the same artichoke dip that we have all come to love, but it is much lighter. Though it is a lighter version, we have been able to improve on the delicious flavor we are all familiar with. It is chuck full of nutritious fat and sodium and perfect as an aside with your vegetables.

Nutritional Information per serving:

Total Carbs: 14.0g; Protein: 17.8g; Fat: 53.9g; Fibre: 2.1g; Sodium: 1,616mg; Calories:643

Ingredients:

- ¼ tbsp. of ground white pepper
- 1 pound of grated parmesan cheese
- 1 finely chopped medium size green bell pepper, seeded and stemmed
- 1 finely chopped medium size red bell pepper, seeded and stemmed
- 2 cups of homemade mayonnaise
- 2 cans of drained and chopped quartered artichoke hearts
- 3 cloves of minced garlic

Directions:

1. Preheat the oven to a temperature of 160 degrees Celsius.

2. Mix all the ingredients in a large bowl, leaving out just ¼ of the parmesan cheese.

3. Spread out the mixed ingredients on a baking dish. Next, sprinkle the parmesan cheese on the mixture.

4. Bake the mixture till it is golden brown; about 45 minutes.

5. Take out of the oven and serve hot.

Plant Based Entrées

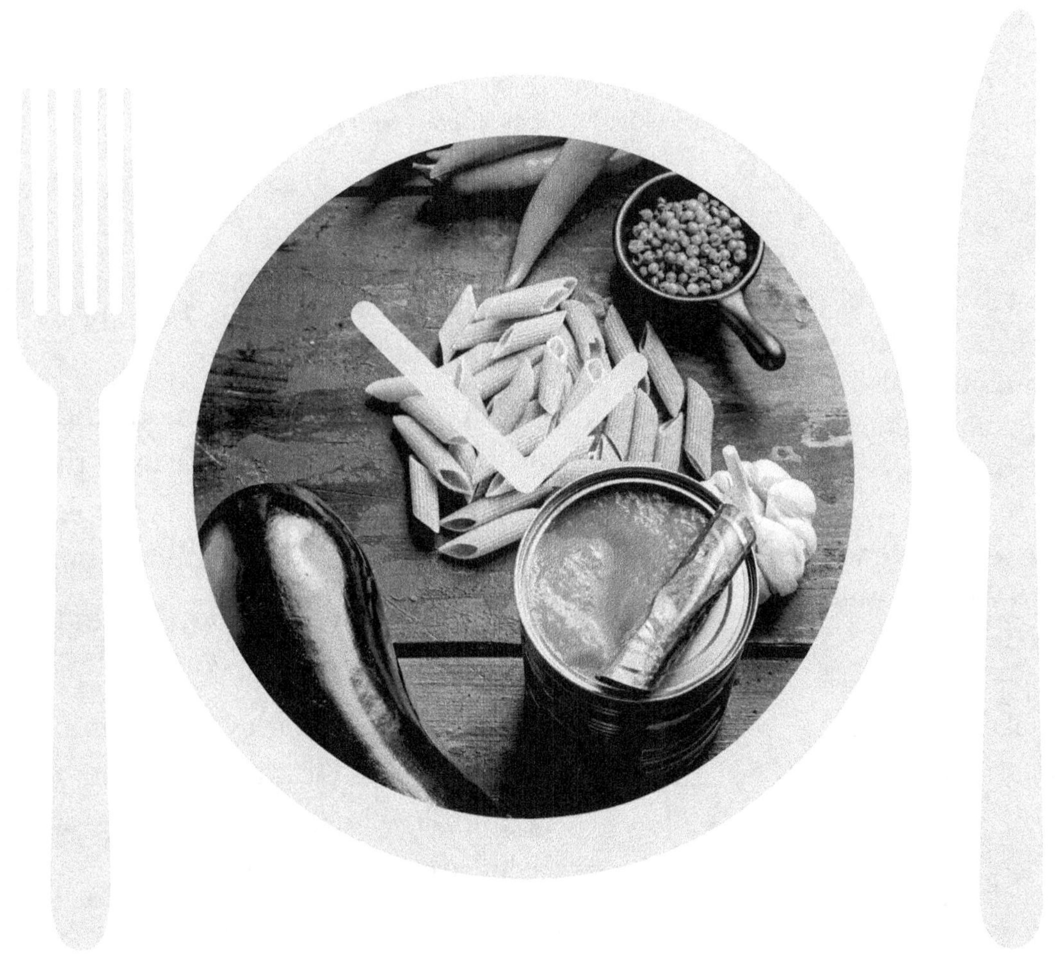

Mushroom Barley Risotto with Chicken

Preparation time: 
55 MINUTES

Cooking time: 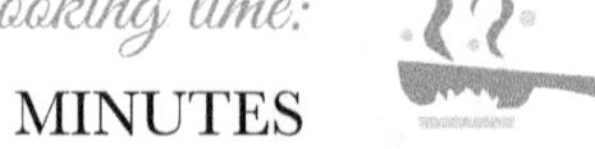
45 MINUTES

Servings: 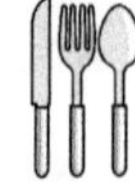
2

The mushroom barley risotto with chicken entrée is definitely one of a kind. This recipe allows you to savor the unique, delectable flavor of mushrooms with spicy flavored chicken. The mushrooms in this entrée are fantastic sources of B Vitamins, which help to prevent a variety of diseases and strengthen the immune systems. The mushrooms also contribute selenium to the body system. Selenium is an important antioxidant that helps to retard the action of free radicals on the body, thereby helping to slow down aging and reduce susceptibility to disease. Mushrooms are low-calorie fungi, meaning that you can have lots of this savory snack without having to worry about piling up calories.

The mushroom barley with risotto chicken takes a total cooking time of forty-five minutes and can be enjoyed as a full, healthy dish.

Nutritional Information per serving:

Calories 600; Total fat: 25g; Saturated fat: 7g; Cholesterol: 30mg; Sodium: 740mg; Carbohydrates: 45g; Fiber: 1g; Sugar: 6g; Protein: 17g.

Ingredients:

- 2 tsp. tablespoon of butter
- 1 lb (450 g) coffee mushrooms, sliced
- One onion, chopped
- Four garlic cloves, finely chopped
- ½ cup dry white wine
- 3 cups 25% less-sodium chicken broth
- 1 cup pearl barley, uncooked
- 1/3 cups Kraft 100% Parmesan Aged Grated Cheese
- 1 cup chopped fresh thyme leaves

Directions:

1. Melt the butter in a large saucepan over medium-high heat.

2. Add in the mushrooms, onion, and garlic and cook for 10 minutes or until the water in the mushrooms is almost completely evaporated. Keep stirring occasionally.

3. Add the wine and cook for 1 minute or until fully absorbed, stirring constantly.

4. Stir in the broth, barley, and thyme and bring to a boil. Cover and simmer on medium-low heat for 45 minutes or until the barley are tender but firm.

5. Remove the risotto from heat.

6. Add the cheese and mix lightly, then serve.

Zucchini-Onion Pizza with Emmental Cheese

Preparation time: 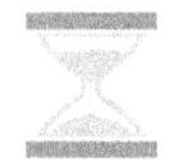
55 MINUTES

Cooking time: 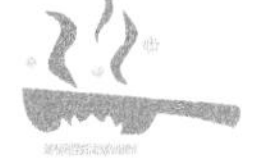
25 MINUTES

Servings: 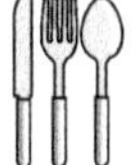
8

If there is one single dish that you'd want to incorporate into your diet to start improving your health right away, it should definitely be the zucchini-onion pizza. This plant-based entrée is fortified with healthy antioxidants that help to control the effects of free radicals, which cause rapid aging. This dish is also filled with fibers to aid digestion, and with its minimal calories, it's a great regular dish to help you lose excess weight. Zucchini can be important in helping to improve long-term cardiac health and can help to regulate natural blood sugar levels. The zucchini-onion pizza may sound a little complicated, but it is actually quite easy to make and can be fully completed in under 2 hours. So, this dish might not be suitable if you want to grab a quick bite, but its unbeatable taste and unrivaled health benefits make it worth the wait.

Nutritional Information per serving:

Calories 570; Total fat: 22g; Saturated fat: 8g; Cholesterol: 40 mg; Sodium: 840mg; Carbohydrates: 64g; Fiber: 1g; Sugar: 13g; Protein: 26g.

Ingredients:

For the dough:
- 300g flour
- 7.5g fresh yeast (or 3.5 g of dehydrated)
- 2 tbsp. olive oil
- 140g lukewarm water
- 1 tsp. of salt

For the garnish:
- Two large white onions
- Two zucchinis
- 10cl fresh cream
- 80g grated Emmental

Directions:

For the dough:

1. Place the flour in a dish, add the water, oil, baking powder, and salt. Gradually stir the mixture to achieve an even consistency until you can press handfuls of the dough into balls.

2. Spread the dough on the work surface and work it for a few minutes (it should not stick), and let it rest for 30 to 40 minutes at room temperature (around 20 ° C). The dough must double in volume.

3. Then, divide the dough in half and spread it 1/2 cm thick on a baking sheet. Let the dough rise again for 25 to 30 minutes.

For the garnish:

1. Peel the onions and cut them into strips, and then wash the zucchinis and cut them into thin slices.

2. Sauté the onions and zucchini until they are brown, and then deglaze with the liquid cream. Stop cooking.

3. Place the filling on the dough, sprinkle with Emmental cheese, and place in the oven. Bake for 15 to 20 minutes at 220 ° C.

4. Serve hot and relish.

Arugula Salad, Cherry Tomatoes, And Pine Nuts

Preparation time:

10 MINUTES

Cooking time:

0 MINUTES

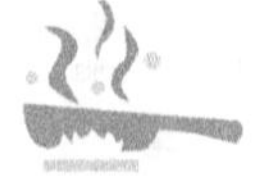

Servings:

4

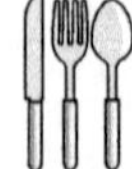

Arugula salad featuring cherry tomatoes and pine nuts is another plant-based entrée that can be relished during intermittent fasting. This particular dish contains arugula, which is rich in calcium, thereby aiding bone and teeth strength and ensuring the normal clotting of blood in the case of physical trauma. Arugula is also a rich store of folate, making it an important vegetable for pregnant women, as folate is essential to fetal development. Folate also contributes to proper growth and tissue building in adults. Arugula also contains vitamin C, which contributes immensely to building immunity, and vitamin K, which further helps to boost arugula's blood-coagulation capabilities. This dish doesn't just feature arugula, however. It also features cherry tomatoes, which are fantastic sources of Vitamin A, which aids clear eyesight, and Vitamin E, which has anti-oxidative properties that help to reduce the effects of aging. The pine nuts in this recipe are abundant sources of calcium and potassium, which both aid bone strength, and dietary fibers that aid digestion.
The arugula salad with cherry tomatoes and pine nuts recipe is very easy to put together. This dish is made from easy-to-source local ingredients and can be fixed in just fifteen minutes.

Nutritional Information per serving:

Calories 610; Total fat: 46g; Saturated fat: 9g; Cholesterol: 20 mg; Sodium: 800mg;
Carbohydrates: 40g; Fiber: 6g; Sugar: 5g; Protein: 17g.

Ingredients:

- 2 tbsp. tablespoons of olive oil
- 1 cup rice vinegar
- ½ tsp. salt
- ¼ tsp. pepper
- 4 cups of arugula leaves
- 1 cup cherry tomatoes, halved
- 1/4 cup pine nuts
- 1/4 cup grated Parmesan
- One large avocado, peeled, pitted, sliced

Directions:

1. Combine the olive oil, vinegar, salt, and pepper in a dish.

2. Place the other ingredients in a bowl and add the vinaigrette.

3. Stir the entire mixture well and garnish with the avocado slices.

Preparation time: 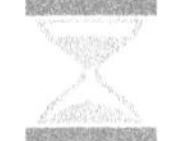 35 MINUTES | **Cooking time:** 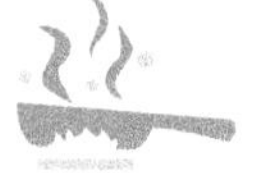 25 MINUTES | **Servings:** 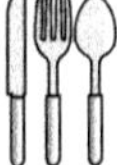 4

Eggplants have always been an abundant source of essential vitamins and minerals, and what better way to balance nutrition and an unbeatable taste than eggplant pasta? You're right, none. Eggplant pasta brings the evergreen fun of pasta together with the powerful health benefits of eggplants and tomatoes. Eggplant pasta is an amazing source of B vitamins which help to prevent a variety of diseases from goiter to pellagra, vitamin D, which helps to improve bone health and prevent rickets, especially in kids, vitamin C which helps to boost immunity and promote the speedy healing of wounds, and Vitamin A which helps to improve eyesight. Eggplant pasta also contains important other important biochemical nutrients that boost cardiac health, reduce an individual's susceptibility to cancers, and improve brain functioning.

Eggplant pasta is pretty convenient to make, can be prepared from locally sourced ingredients, and cooks in just twenty minutes.

Nutritional Information per serving:

Calories 249; Total fat: 13 g; Saturated fat: 2 g; Cholesterol: 0 mg; Sodium: 364 mg; Carbohydrates: 32g; Fiber: 5g; Sugar: 5g; Protein: 6g.

Ingredients:

Pasta
- 500 g of pasta
- Tomato coulis
- 50 cl of tomato coulis or tomato puree

Eggplant
- One eggplant, diced
- Two large tomatoes cut into cubes.
- 5 tbsp. extra virgin olive oil
- 4 tbsp. Veal broth
- One clove of garlic
- 1 tbsp. balsamic vinegar
- Two fresh basil leaves
- ½ tsp. Chili powder
- ½ tsp. Salt
- ¼ tsp. Ground pepper.
- 1 tsp. Parmesan cheese.

Directions:

1. Cook the pasta as indicated on the package.

2. Put the eggplants to cook in a pan with olive oil, salt, and pepper. Heat till the eggplants get golden-brown in color and then set aside.

3. Cut the cherry tomatoes in half and cook over high heat in the pan. Add in the chopped garlic cloves and the balsamic vinegar.

4. Add the veal broth into the tomato sauce and season with salt and pepper. Simmer over low heat for 3-4 minutes.

5. Return the eggplants to the sauce and add the basil. Cook for 1 minute, just enough time to reheat the eggplants.

6. Add the drained pasta to the sauce, simmer for 1 or 2 minutes and serve immediately. Sprinkle with Parmesan and enjoy!

Zucchini Boats and Carrots

35 MINUTES 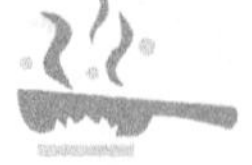

20 MINUTES

2 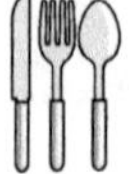

Zucchini boats and carrots give a whole new meaning to healthy, adventurous eating. Zucchini boats are a classic vegetarian favorite, and they are incredibly perfect for intermittent fasting purposes. Zucchinis are fortified with most of the essential vitamins the body needs to function optimally; Vitamin A for great eyesight, vitamin C for strengthening your immunity and improving wound healing capabilities, and Vitamin K for efficient blood clotting. Zucchinis are also great sources of potassium, which helps to keep blood pressure levels stable and healthy and helping to reduce the risks of hypertension and cardiac complications.

Carrots, on the other hand, are famous for being rich sources of vitamin A which enhances optimal eyesight. Carrots are also brilliant sources of potassium and manganese, making them important for the enhanced functioning of the body's central nervous systems. Carrots are also great sources of antioxidants, which help to reduce the effects of aging and reduce the susceptibility of the body to age-related diseases. Carrots and zucchinis are both low-calorie foods, making this uniquely delicious dish an amazing one for people concerned about weight gain.

Zucchini boats stuffed with carrots cook in about forty minutes can be enjoyed at any time of the day, and are made from locally sourced ingredients.

Nutritional Information per serving:

Calories 470; Total fat: 25g; Saturated fat: 7g; Cholesterol: 30mg; Sodium: 740mg; Carbohydrates: 45g; Fiber: 1g; Sugar: 6g; Protein: 17g.

Ingredients:

- 75g ham
- One egg
- Chopped onions
- Two large carrots
- One zucchini

Directions:

1. Preheat the oven to 180 °. Wash and cut the zucchini in half lengthwise. Hollow them out with a spoon, keep the flesh. Place the dish with the empty zucchinis in the oven for about ten minutes.

2. Meanwhile, in the bowl of a food processor, put the zucchini flesh, onion, carrots cut into large pieces, and ham. Coarsely chop, it should not be too fine.

3. Brown the mince in a pan for about ten minutes.

4. Beat the egg and add it to the pan to bind the whole. Stir quickly, then stop cooking.

5. Take the dish out of the oven and garnish the zucchini with the stuffing, bake for about twenty minutes and enjoy!

Seafood Entrées

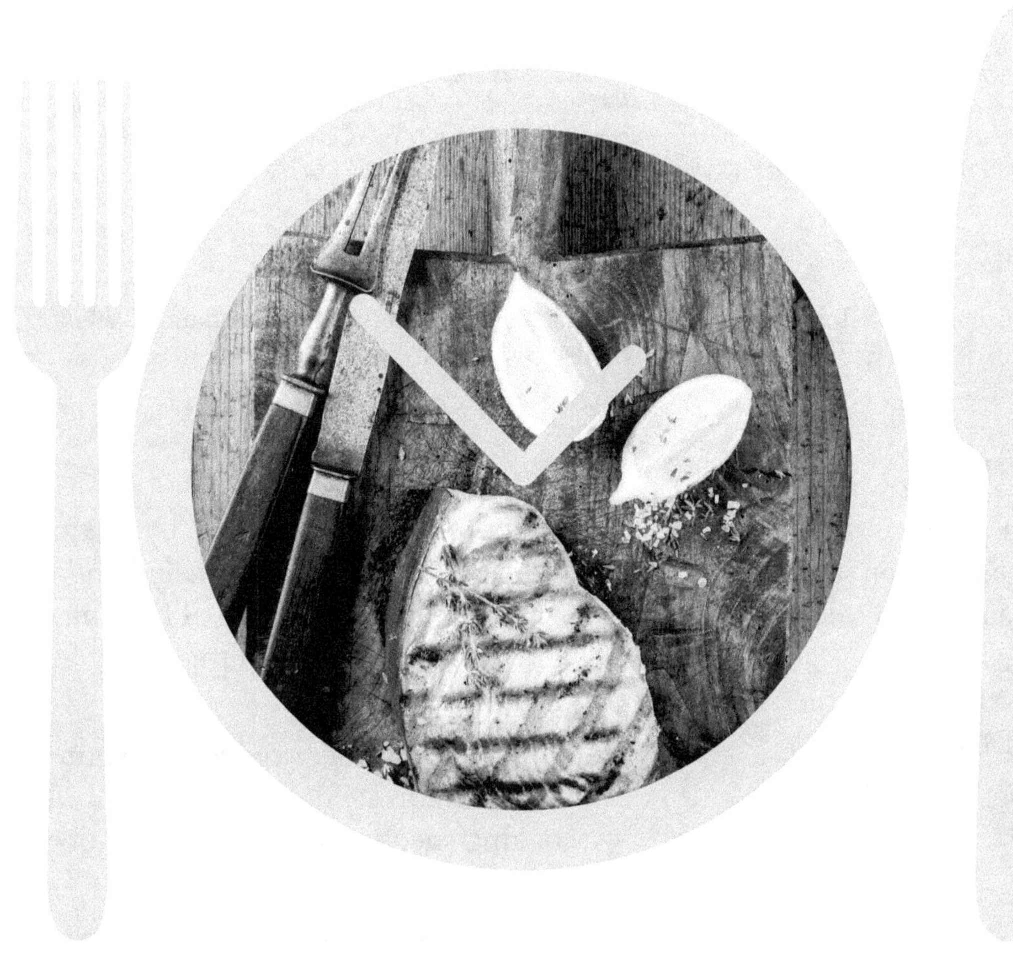

Teriyaki Salmon Steak

40 MINUTES

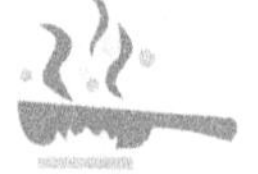

20 MINUTES

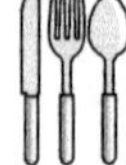

4

The teriyaki salmon steak is an exquisite exotic dish that allows you to enjoy the distinctive taste of salmon in the best way possible—like a steak. Salmon are reputable for being excellent sources of essential Omega 3 Fatty acids, which have a wide variety of health benefits that are treasured by health-conscious individuals all over the globe. The omega-3 fatty acids that are abundant in salmon can help to fight depression and anxiety and lead to all-round better mental health and emotional stability. Omega-3 fatty acids are also extremely potent at enhancing eyesight and can help to reduce your susceptibility to cardiac complications in the long run. Pregnant women are especially advised to consume high amounts of Omega-3 fatty acids as they help to ensure proper nervous system development of the baby.

Salmon also contains a number of other important bioactive compounds such as protective antioxidants that help to reduce the health effects of aging and retard the action of harmful free radicals. Salmon is also a rich source of essential B vitamins and potassium, and selenium, which are key in maintaining optimal immunity levels and reducing susceptibility to diseases. The teriyaki salmon steak is delightfully delicious, appropriate for all kinds of occasions, and cooks in barely 20 minutes.

Nutritional Information per serving:

Calories 310; Total fat: 15g; Saturated fat: 4 g; Cholesterol: 55 mg; Sodium: 1230 mg; Carbohydrates: 16g; Fiber: 0g; Sugar: 12g; Protein: 25g.

Ingredients:

- 4 Salmon fillets
- 3tbsp. tablespoon soy sauce
- 3tbsp. Japanese cooking sake
- 3tbsp. Mirin (rice wine)
- 2cm of ginger root
- 0.5tbsp. tablespoon Sugar
- Sesame seeds

Directions:

1. Prepare the teriyaki sauce by mixing the soy sauce, mirin, sake, and peeled and finely grated ginger in a bowl. The salmon steaks are to be marinated in this sauce for 20 minutes.

2. Preheat the broiler section of your oven. The salmon steaks should be transferred to a baking sheet and cooked at 400 degrees for 15 minutes.

3. Heat the sauce and add the sugar while stirring. As soon as the sugar is fully melted, brush the salmon fillets with the thickened sauce and heat a few minutes under the grill.

4. Sprinkle the salmon steaks with sesame seeds, garnish with lemon wedges, and serve hot.

Vibrant Veggie Shrimp Stir-Fry with Cashews and Egg Roll Fried Rice

Preparation time: 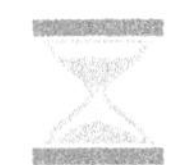

25 MINUTES

Cooking time: 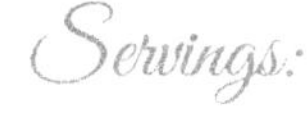

10 MINUTES

Servings: 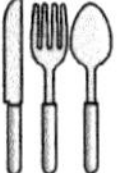

2

This is a combination of two dishes that come with color and flavor. Even though this dishes can be enjoyed separately, it is heavenly to eat them together.

Nutritional Information per serving:

28g of protein, 35g of Fat, 25.9g of Net Carbs, 1358mg of Sodium, 932 mg of Potassium, 536 Calories

Ingredients:

For the Stir-Fry
- Salt and black pepper
- 1 tbsp. of minced garlic
- 1 tbsp. of neutral tasting oil
- 8 ounces of peeled raw shrimps
- 1 cup of bit-sized broccoli florets pieces
- 1 cup of trimmed and de-threaded snow peas
- 2 tbsp. of tamari or coconut amino
- ½ cup of cashew

For the Egg Roll Fried Rice
- ½ cup of shredded green cabbage
- 1 tbsp. of minced garlic
- 1 tbsp. of neutral flavored oil
- ½ cup of shredded carrot
- 2 green onions separated into finely chopped white and greens
- Salt
- 1 egg
- 1 tbsp. of tamari or coconut amino
- 1 cup of cooked white rice or cauliflower rice
- 2 tbsp. of minced fresh garlic
- ½ tbsp. of sesame oil

Directions:

How to make the stir-fry;
1. Use salt and pepper to season the shrimps lightly.
2. Heat oil in a pan on high heat until the oil flows freely. Put in the broccoli, shrimps, and snow peas.
3. Fry for two minutes while stirring from time to time. Add garlic, ginger, and cashews.
4. Mix well and cook for two to three minutes until the shrimps become completely opaque and the garlic and ginger are becoming brown.
5. Gently stir in the tamari or coconut amino. Transfer the mixture to a dish and cover to keep it warm.

How to make the rice;
1. Rinse the frying pan and place it on medium-high heat.
2. Let the pot dry and become warm. Add oil and allow it to shimmer. Add carrot, cabbage, garlic, ginger, a pinch of salt, and the white parts of green onions.
3. Mix well and let it cook for five minutes. Stir frequently as it cooks, and do not allow the ginger and garlic to go brown.
4. Add rice and sesame oil when the garlic becomes almost translucent and soft. Cook for another three minutes.
5. In the center of the mixture, create a well. Crack the egg in and break the yolk immediately. Let it cook for thirty seconds and blend it with the rest of the mixture.
6. Stir in 1 tbsp. of tamari or coconut amino. Remove from heat.
7. Serve the fried rice and stir-fry on two plates and garnish with the green parts of the green onions.

Grilled Swordfish

Preparation time: 20 MINUTES   **Cooking time:** 15 MINUTES 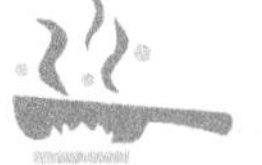   **Servings:** 4 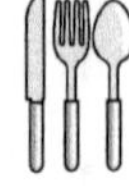

Grilled swordfish is another uniquely tasty food on the intermittent fasting menu with mind-blowing health benefits. Swordfish is a naturally powerful source of selenium, making it significant in the prevention of cancer and cardiac complications. Swordfish is also rich in proteins, which function in tissue building and cellular repair; zinc, which boosts the functioning of the immune system; and omega-3 fatty acids, which aid excellent eyesight, promote optimal brain health, and ensure excellent fetal development. Grilled swordfish is also a rich source of niacin, an essential nutrient lacking in most of today's modern diets. Niacin can also help to lower unhealthy cholesterol and saturated fats levels, thereby helping to reduce the risk of obesity and its related complications such as cardiac disease. Niacin also plays an important role in helping to regulate blood sugar levels, thereby reducing susceptibility to type-1-diabetes. Niacin is also essential to optimum brain function, healthy skin, and strong bones.

Grilled swordfish is not just nutritious and exciting; it's fun to cook, can be prepared for locally-sourced materials, and is an excellent dish for any occasion.

Nutritional Information per serving:

Calories 395; Total fat: 27g; Saturated fat: 5 g; Cholesterol: 66 mg; Sodium: 294 mg; Carbohydrates: 3g; Fiber: 0g; Sugar: 1g; Protein: 34g.

Ingredients:

- Four thin slices of swordfish
- One clove of garlic
- One lemon
- Five sprigs of fresh curly parsley
- 3 tbsp. Extra virgin olive oil
- ½ tsp. Salt
- ¼ tsp. freshly ground pepper

Directions:

1. Peel and finely chop the garlic.
2. Clean and pat dry the fresh parsley and cut it into pieces.
3. Cut the lemon in half and squeeze it to collect its juice.
4. Heat the olive oil in a pan over medium heat.
5. When the olive oil is hot, add the chopped garlic and chopped parsley and sauté for 1 minute, until golden brown.
6. Place the swordfish slices in the pan and cook for 2 minutes on each side.
7. Deglaze the pan by pouring in the lemon juice, then add salt and pepper to taste. Leave to cook for a few more minutes over low heat.
8. Arrange the swordfish slices on the plates and top them with the lemon juice sauce.
9. Serve immediately with rice, fresh tagliatelle, or a nice homemade mashed potato.

Mediterranean Baked Shrimp

Preparation time: 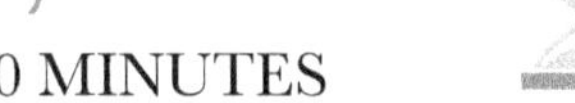
20 MINUTES

Cooking time: 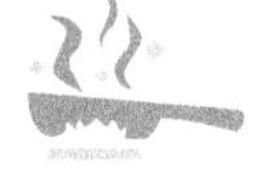
12 MINUTES

Servings: 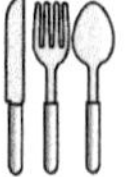
4

The baked shrimp is forever a rave winning meal when it comes to reviews. It is fast and simple to bake shrimps. With the zing and flavor from nutrient-packed thyme and oregano, the baked shrimp can't get any better.

Nutritional Information per serving:

In one serving, you get 21 g of protein, 11 g of Fat, 3.6g of Net Carbs, 857 mg of Sodium, 230 mg of Potassium, and 199 Calories.

Ingredients:

- Zest of 1 lemon
- 2 tbsp. of extra virgin olive oil
- 1 pound of peeled, deveined, fresh or thawed shrimp
- ½ tbsp. of fresh or lemon thyme
- 1 tbsp. of fresh oregano
- Black pepper and salt for taste

Directions:

1. Use parchment paper to line a baking tray. Preheat the oven to 400 degrees Fahrenheit.

2. Mix all the ingredients well in a medium bowl and toss very well until the shrimps are well coated.

3. Place the coated shrimps in straight lines on the parchment paper. Move it into the oven. Bake for ten to twelve minutes until the shrimps become firm. Ensure that the shrimps are not translucent along their thickest parts. Serve and enjoy.

Basic Baked Scallops

Preparation time: 

25 MINUTES

Cooking time: 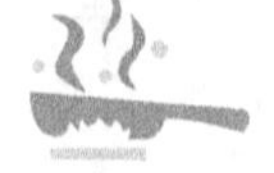

14 MINUTES

Servings: 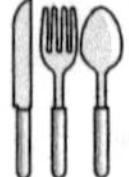

1

Thirty minutes is all it takes to prepare this delicious seafood recipe. It goes really well with salad or green beans, depending on your preference.

Nutritional Information per serving:

Total Carbs: 13.4g; Protein: 26.8g; Fat: 42.7g; Fibre: 3.5g; Sodium: 907mg; Calories:540

Ingredients:

- ¼ tbsp. of sea salt
- ½ tbsp. of smoked paprika
- ½ cup of almond meal
- ½ tbsp. of freshly ground black pepper
- 2 tbsp. of freshly squeezed lemon juice
- 2 tbsp. of Olive Oil
- 2 tbsp. of fresh flat-leaf parsley, chopped
- 2 ½ tbsp. of melted grass-fed butter, unsalted
- ¾ pound of sea scallops

Directions:

1. Preheat the oven to a temperature of 220 degrees Celsius.

2. Get a baking dish. Pour in the butter, salt, pepper, lemon juice, and scallops. Toss them together.

3. In a separate bowl, mix the olive oil, almond meal, parsley, and paprika together. Sprinkle this mix on the scallops in the baking dish.

4. Bake the scallops in the oven till the almond meal turns golden; this would take about 14 minutes. Remove from the oven and serve immediately.

Sautéed Branzino

Preparation time: 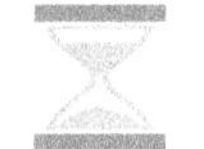

30 MINUTES

Cooking time: 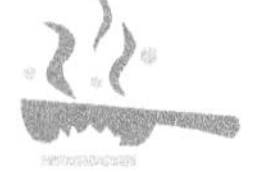

20 MINUTES

Servings: 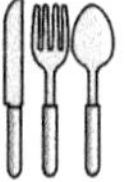

4

Sautéed branzino is a simple yet exceptional dish that consists primarily of the exotic branzino fish. Branzino is a powerhouse of important biochemical nutrients, from proteins that help in bodybuilding to Vitamin D that improves bone density and immunity while helping to reduce susceptibility in rickets, especially in young children. Branzino fish is also an excellent source of Omega-3 fatty acids, which are important in boosting immunity, promoting optimal brain health, and boosting fetal development.

Nutritional Information per serving:

Calories 432; Total fat: 25g; Saturated fat: 4 g; Cholesterol: 70 mg; Sodium: 231 mg; Carbohydrates: 13g; Fiber: 4g; Sugar: 1g; Protein: 37g.

Ingredients:

- Four pieces of branzino fish
- Two cloves garlic
- Two tomatoes
- Two onions
- 3 tbsp. extra virgin olive oil
- One lemon
- 1 tbsp. Parsley
- ½ tsp. Salt
- ¼ tsp. pepper

Directions:

1. Peel the onions and garlic, then mince them.
2. Cut the lemon into large slices and the tomato into quarters.
3. Roughly chop the parsley.
4. Oil the bottom of the baking sheet. Arrange the tomatoes then the branzino fillets
5. Garnish the fish with lemon, parsley, garlic, onion. Add in salt and pepper.
6. Drizzle with olive oil.
7. Preheat the oven to 180/200 ° C, then cook for about 20 minutes.

Bright Coriander Roasted Salmon

20 MINUTES 

11 MINUTES 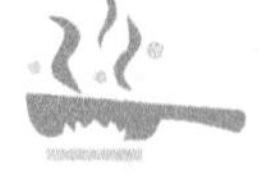

2 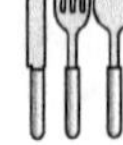

Not only is it really quick to make, but Salmond is also almost a nutritious food for any time.

Nutritional Information per serving:

In one serving, you get 29 g of protein, 21 g of Fat, 0.3g of Net Carbs, 85 mg of Sodium, 532 mg of Potassium, and 318 Calories.

Ingredients:

- 10 ounces of Salmon
- 2 tbsp. of lemon juice
- ½ tbsp. pf ground coriander
- 1 tbsp. of extra virgin olive oil
- ½ tbsp. of coriander seeds
- ½ tbsp. of lemon zests
- Black pepper and salt for taste

Directions:

1. Use parchment paper to line a pie tin and preheat the oven to 425 degrees Fahrenheit

2. Cut the salmon into two fillets on parchment paper. Season the fillets with pepper and salt and set them aside.

3. Whisk the lemon juice, ground coriander, lemon zest, and olive oil together in a bowl. Distribute the mixture evenly over the salmon fillets. Sprinkle coriander seeds on top.

4. Bake the fillets for eleven minutes and serve.

Roasted Cauliflower

 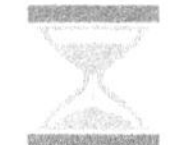

1 H 35 MINUTES

 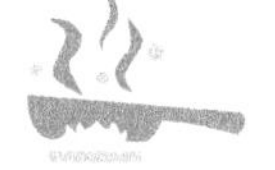

1 H 20 MINUTES

 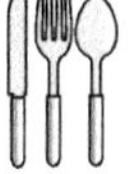

5

Roasted cauliflower is a relatively uncommon dish with exceptional nutritional properties. Cauliflower is reputed for being a rich source of sulforaphane, an organic derivative of sulfur that helps to reduce internal inflammations and reduce the susceptibility of individuals to cancers. Sulforaphane also plays an active role in liver detoxification. The liver plays an essential role in helping to metabolize toxic substances and drugs that would otherwise be harmful to the body. Consuming cauliflower helps to remove deposits of toxic materials found in the liver.

Cauliflower is also reputed to improve cardiac health, promote healthy brain function, and promote a healthy hormonal balance. Roasted cauliflower can be easily prepared in a little over an hour, can be prepared from locally-sourced ingredients, and is perfect for vegetarians.

Nutritional Information per serving:

Calories 110; Total fat: 7g; Saturated fat: 1g; Cholesterol: 0 mg; Sodium: 130mg;
Carbohydrates: 10g; Fiber: 3g; Sugar: 4g; Protein: 3g.

Ingredients:

- One cabbage leaf
- 3 tbsp. olive oil
- Two pinches of fleur de sel (sea salt)
- ½ tsp. freshly ground pepper
- Three garlic cloves, chopped
- 1 tbsp. parsley

Tahina sauce

- 3 tbsp. tahini
- 50cl lemon juice
- 50cl Water
- ½ tsp. Salt
- ¼ tsp. ground pepper
- One clove of garlic
- 1 tbsp. chopped parsley

Directions:

1. Preheat the oven to 200 ° C. Cut off the larger leaves from the cauliflower. Cut the stem off at the base so that the cauliflower stands upright. Wash the cauliflower thoroughly and allow it to dry a bit.

2. Place the cauliflower on a baking sheet lined with parchment paper. Brush the cauliflower with olive oil, season with salt and pepper. Wrap it entirely with baking paper (this will prevent it from darkening at its base). Bake for about 1 hour or until the cauliflower is tender when you prick it.

3. Remove the cauliflower from the oven. In a small bowl, combine two tablespoons of olive oil with the chopped garlic cloves and parsley and pour over the cauliflower. Bake for another 20 minutes uncovered this time.

4. Right out of the oven, serve immediately and sprinkle with a little chopped parsley. You can serve this roasted cauliflower with a small sauce composed of tahini (sesame paste), salt, pepper, lemon juice, parsley, and a little garlic.

Roasted Brussels Sprouts

Preparation time: 20 MINUTES

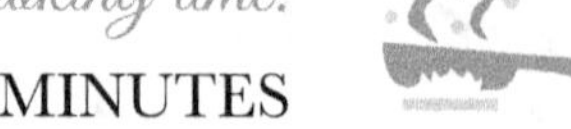

Cooking time: 10 MINUTES

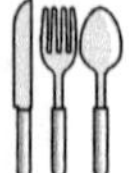

Servings: 6

Roasted Brussels Sprouts are perfect if you are looking for a different, novel kind of excitement while keeping things healthy and nutritious. Brussels sprouts are rich sources of fiber, aiding easy digestion. Brussels sprouts are also rich in vitamins, minerals, and antioxidants, thereby helping to strengthen the immune system and reduce susceptibility to dangerous diseases. Brussels sprouts, if consumed in the long-term, have been found to reduce the risks of cancer, diabetes, and inflammations.
This particular recipe combines roasted brussels sprouts with bacon and mustard, can be cooked within half an hour and is absolutely perfect for a variety of occasions.

Nutritional Information per serving:

Calories 113; Total fat: 7g; Saturated fat: 1g; Cholesterol: 0mg; Sodium: 174mg; Carbohydrates: 11g; Fiber: 4g; Sugar: 3g; Protein: 4g.

Ingredients:

- Three slices of bacon, finely diced
- 1 tbsp. Olive oil
- 6 cups Brussels sprouts (halved)
- ¾-cup chicken broth or apple juice
- 1 tbsp. Old-fashioned mustard
- ½ tsp. Salt
- ¼ tsp. ground pepper

Directions:

1. In a large non-stick skillet over medium-high heat, heat the bacon in the oil. Remove the bacon with a skimmer. Reserve on a plate. Keep the fat in the pan.

2. In the same skillet, brown the sprouts in the hot fat, and add salt and pepper. Deglaze with the broth and mustard. Bring to a boil and simmer over medium heat for 10 minutes or until the sprouts are tender and the broth has evaporated, stirring frequently. Adjust seasoning.

3. Transfer to a serving dish and sprinkle with bacon.

Sesame Broccoli

Preparation time: 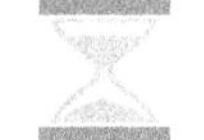
15 MINUTES

Cooking time: 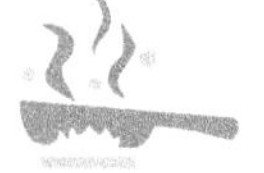
10 MINUTES

Servings: 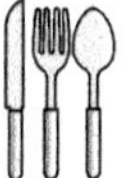
4

Sesame broccoli is a simple, easy-to-cook intermittent fasting recipe that can be enjoyed at any time of the day. This dish can be made under 15 minutes of total preparation time, and for such a quick dish, it tastes incredible. Broccoli is a rich source of fiber which aids digestion, and proteins which function in building tissue and enhancing cellular repair. Broccoli is also an abundant source of iron, which promotes the formation of red blood cells, thereby ensuring optimal blood circulation and preventing anemia. Broccoli also contains potassium, which aids in exceptional brain function, calcium that ensures optimal bone density, and the essential vitamins that help to strengthen the immune system while preventing a wide variety of specific diseases.

Nutritional Information per serving:

Calories 92; Total fat: 1g; Saturated fat: 1g; Cholesterol: 0mg; Sodium: 112mg; Carbohydrates: 5g; Fiber: 3g; Sugar: 1g; Protein: 4g.

Ingredients:

- One broccoli, cut into florets and blanched
- 1 tbsp. Vegetable oil
- 1 tsp. Sesame oil
- 2 tsp. Sesame seeds
- ½ tsp. Salt
- ¼ tsp. pepper

Directions:

1. Heat the vegetable oil over medium hit in a non-stick skillet, and sauté the broccoli for 2 minutes.

2. Add in the salt, pepper, sesame oil, and sesame seeds

3. Allow to cook properly, and serve hot.

Preparation time: 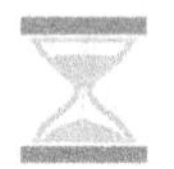

20 MINUTES

Cooking time: 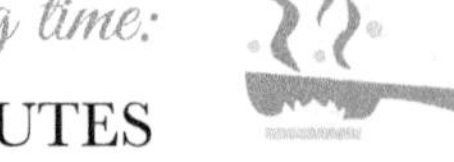

14 MINUTES

Servings: 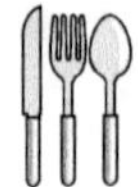

4

Organic quinoa with roasted nuts is perhaps one of the most nutritionally beneficial and simple foods to make in the intermittent fasting recipe recommendations. Quinoa is a highly nutritious food option containing the natural plant compounds Quercetin and Kaempferol, which are specialized compounds that aid in weight loss and supply the body with essential antioxidants that repress the activities of harmful free radicals derived from the regular foods we eat. Quinoa is higher in fiber than most grains, meaning that it would aid easy digestion and improve gut health. Quinoa also has a very low gluten content and is high in protein instead, further making it a great option for people looking to lose weight and maintain a healthy muscle mass. Quinoa also has a low glycemic index, making it important in the regulation of blood sugar levels.

The roasted nuts to be used in this recipe include almonds, macadamia nuts, and cashew. These nuts combine to give a healthy combination that supplies the body with considerable amounts of fiber, monosaturated fats, proteins, and Vitamin E, which is essential for an optimal immune system function. Quinoa with roasted nuts can be put together in less than thirty minutes and can be made from cheap, locally-sourced ingredients.

Nutritional Information per serving:

Calories 194; Total fat: 8g; Saturated fat: 1.5g; Cholesterol: 0 mg; Sodium: 192mg; Carbohydrates: 26g; Fiber: 3g; Sugar: 4g; Protein: 7g.

Ingredients:

- 2 cups of organic quinoa
- 2 cups cashew, macadamia, and almond mixture
- 1 Lemon
- One garlic clove, minced
- 1 cup flat-leaf parsley
- ½ cup dill
- ½ cup basil leaves
- 1 cup of coriander leaves
- ½ cup mint leaves
- 2 tbsp. olive oil
- ½ tsp. pepper
- ¼ tsp. salt

Directions:

1. In a colander, rinse the quinoa in cold water until the water runs clear. Pour it into a pot of salted boiling water and stir. Cook it for about 10 minutes until the seeds burst open.

2. Crush the dried fruits and toast them in the oven at (180 ° C for 4 minutes.

3. Combine the peeled and chopped garlic, olive oil, lemon zest, and juice, one pinch of salt and pepper in a bowl.

4. When the quinoa is cooked, drain it and rinse it with water to cool it a bit. Mix the quinoa with the other ingredients and adjust the seasoning.

5. Rinse and roughly chop the herbs and add them just before serving.

Steak and Sweet Potato Fries

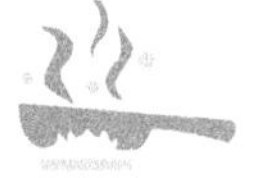

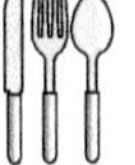

When talking about exquisite American classics, steak and fries are undisputed kings. Steak is an excellent source of protein, which is critical to tissue building and cellular regeneration. Steak is also an important source of iron, which aids in the synthesis of new red blood cells that function in circulation. Steak has also been proven to reduce incidences of mental fog, thereby helping to enhance clarity and long-term mental health.

Potatoes, on the other hand, are excellent sources of vitamin A, which enhances eyesight and prevents the early onset of ocular degeneration. Potatoes can also help to reduce an individual's chances of contracting Type-1 diabetes by aiding in blood sugar regulation. Potatoes can also play critical roles in helping to relieve stress and helping individuals feel more energetic, as they are concentrated carbohydrate sources. Regular consumption of potatoes has also been proven to aid in the prevention of inflammations, cancer, ulcers, and cardiovascular diseases.

Steak and potato fries are unforgettably delicious, appropriate for most occasions, and can be prepared within one hour.

Nutritional Information per serving:

Calories 170; Total fat: 7g; Saturated fat: 1.5g; Cholesterol: 0 mg; Sodium: 615mg; Carbohydrates: 26g; Fiber: 4g; Sugar: 5g; Protein: 2g.

Ingredients:

Mayonnaise Mix
- ½ cup Mayonnaise
- 4 tsp. Prepared mustard
- ½ tsp. Curry powder

Sweet Potato Fries
- Three sweet potatoes, peeled and cut into large spirals.
- ½ cup potato starch
- 5 tbsp. olive oil

Steaks
- 3 tbsp. Pine nuts
- 1 tbsp. Sesame seeds
- 3 tbsp. Olive oil
- 1 tsp. Ground turmeric
- 1 ½ lb. flank steak (or steak), cut into four steaks

Directions:

Mayonnaise Mix
In a bowl, mix all the ingredients. Reserve.

Sweet Potato Fries
1. Preheat the oil in the fryer to 180 ° C (350 ° F). Line a baking sheet with paper towels.
2. Immerse the sweet potato sticks in the water and let them soak for 5 minutes. Drain the potatoes well, then spread them out on the baking sheet. Sprinkle with the potato starch and coat well.
3. Fry a quarter of the sweet potatoes at a time, 3 to 4 minutes, or until lightly browned and crispy. Watch out for splashing. Drain the fries on paper towels and add salt and pepper. Reserve on a baking sheet in an oven preheated to 95 ° C (200 ° F).

Steaks
1. In a large non-stick skillet over medium heat, brown the pine nuts and sesame in 1 tbsp of the oil. Remove from fire. Add the turmeric. Coat the nuts and sesame well. Transfer to a small bowl and set aside.
2. In the same skillet over medium-high heat, brown the meat in the remaining oil for 3 minutes per side for rare doneness: salt and pepper. Let the meat rest on a plate for 5 minutes.
3. Divide a dash of mayonnaise between the plates. Top with the meat and garnish with the pine nut mixture. Serve with sweet potato fries and the rest of the mayonnaise.

Desserts and Snacks

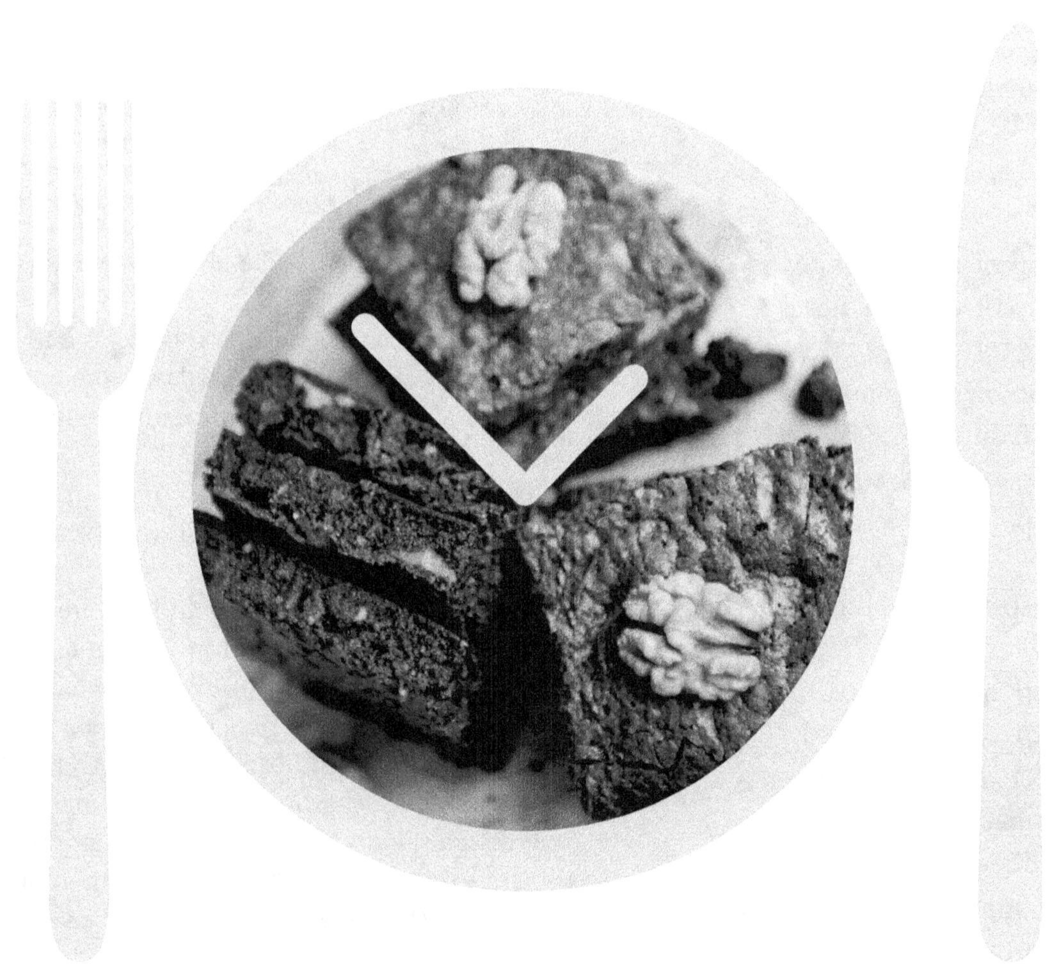

High Protein Vegan Crackers

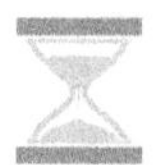

1 HOUR

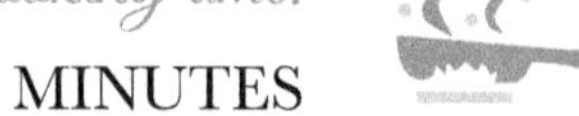

40 MINUTES

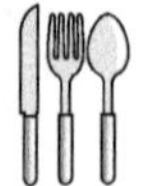

6

These are cakey crackers that do not come with the crumbly feels of a cake. They can be taken in quite a few ways, either dipped into a luscious soup or syrup or topped with meats and cheese. This meal is low in carbs and moderately rich in protein and fat. It is a completely plant-based meal.

Nutritional Information

13g of protein, 14g of Fat, 4g of Net Carbs, 178mg of Sodium, 238mg of Potassium, and 193 Calories.

Ingredients:

- ½ cup of almond flour
- ¼ cup of coconut flour
- ½ cup of water
- ½ cup of hemp protein (unflavoured)
- 3 tbsp. of flaxseed meal
- 1 tbsp. of melted coconut oil
- ¼ tbsp. of fine Himalayan salt
- 1 tbsp. of chia seeds
- 3 tbsp. of sesame seeds
- ¼ tbsp. of garlic powder, paprika, rosemary, chili powder, cumin, caraway seed, and herbs de Provence (all optional as seasoning)

Directions:

1. Place a rack in the middle of an oven and preheat it to 350 Fahrenheit.
2. Get a parchment paper that is twice as long as the baking tray. This will be folded over the crackers.
3. Whisk water and flaxseed meal in a small bowl and set the mixture aside.
4. Mix all the dry ingredients in a medium bowl. Include the seasonings and still well with a fork until the mixture is well blended.
5. Add the mixture from step 3 and coconut oil to the bowl in step 4 and mix thoroughly until a ball is formed. Ensure it is not crumbly but pliable.
6. Spread the parchment paper on an even flat surface and place the dough near the center. Gently fold the paper along its length until the edges meet. Flatten the dough slightly by pressing down on it. Roll the dough to a 9 by 12-inch rectangle with a thickness of about 1/8 inch and cut off the top layer of the parchment paper.
7. Using a knife, cut the dough into six strips. Cut each strip into eight crackers.
8. Bake the crackers for thirty minutes. Next, remove the tray and flip the crackers. Bake for another ten minutes. Remove the crackers from the oven. Allow them to cool well. The crackers can stay for ten days without refrigeration.

Dark Chocolate Brownies and Walnuts

Preparation time: 
35 MINUTES

Cooking time: 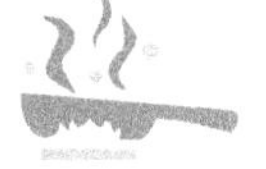
25 MINUTES

Servings: 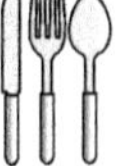
8

Even while trying to stay healthy through intermittent fasting, it is still important to have some exciting food that takes your taste buds on a novel adventure. Chocolates have earned a reputation for having high fat and cholesterol levels. However, dark chocolates are a safer and more nutritious form of chocolate that can actually help you to achieve your calorie-control and weight loss goals if eaten in controlled amounts.

Dark chocolates are powerful sources of antioxidants that can help to offset the effects of damaging free radicals in the body. They have also been found to lower body cholesterol levels, thereby helping to improve blood flow, lower blood pressure, and reduce an individual's risks of contracting cardiac complications in the long-term. Dark chocolates are also excellent for glowing, healthy skin that remains unaffected by ultraviolet rays from the sun.

Walnuts, on the other hand, the second major component of this recipe, are reputed for being rich brain-foods. Walnuts contain important phytochemicals that improve brain health, mental clarity and reduce the rate of brain cell degeneration. Walnuts are also great for boosting your mood, enhancing weight loss, and their high fiber content ensures a healthier and more effective digestive system.

Dark chocolate brownies with walnuts are delicious and undoubtedly great for your health, can be used as a snack or as dessert after the main meal, and can be prepared in under 40 minutes.

Nutritional Information per serving:

Calories 240; Total fat: 17g; Saturated fat: 4g; Cholesterol: 30mg; Sodium: 65mg; Carbohydrates: 21g; Fiber: 2g; Sugar: 13g; Protein: 4g.

Ingredients:

- 200g chocolate
- 125g butter
- 150g sugar
- 70g flour
- 150g walnuts
- Three eggs

Directions:

1. Place the butter in a mold and heat in the oven at 150 ° C to melt the butter.

2. In a salad bowl, pour melted butter and sugar. Mix with a whisk until you obtain a smooth paste.

3. Add eggs and flour and Stir again.

4. Heat the chocolate at 200°C to completely melt it, and then add in the walnuts. Pour the preparation into the mold and bake for 25 minutes at 150 ° C.

Angel Cake

<table>
<tr><td>

4 HOURS

</td><td>

50 MINUTES

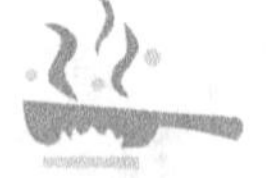</td><td>

6-8

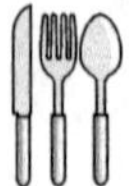</td></tr>
</table>

Angel cake is such an essential component of the intermittent fasting list of recipes because it gives you the opportunity to cure your cravings for calorie and cholesterol-heavy foods using a healthier and more nutritious alternative. Angel cake has been specially formulated to remove the excess calories, fats, and cholesterol that characterize most cakes. This makes angel cake a delicious and fun food, which, when eating in controlled amounts, can also help you to lose weight fast and gain essential nutrients needed for optimal functioning.

However, care must still be taken when eating angel cake, as it still has relatively high sugar content. Angel cake is a rich store of sodium, which enables proper nervous system functioning. The cake also contains calcium, which enhances the clotting of blood when the body suffers physical trauma and promotes strong, healthy bones and teeth. Angel cake also contains considerable amounts of iron, which enables the formation of red blood cells, ensuring proper blood circulation.

The cake is pretty easy to bake, it is made from easy-to-source ingredients and can be completed and savored within one hour.

Nutritional Information per serving:

Calories 131; Total fat: 7g; Saturated fat: 2g; Cholesterol: 13 mg; Sodium: 218mg; Carbohydrates: 26g; Fiber: 0g; Sugar: 15g; Protein: 2g.

Ingredients:

Cake

- One ¼ cups pastry flour
- 1 cup icing sugar
- 1/4 tsp. salt
- 12 egg whites, at room temperature
- 1 tsp. Cream of tartar
- ½ tsp. vanilla extract
- 1 cup granulated sugar

Icing

- 500 ml (2 cups) 35% cream
- 1/4 cup (60 ml) icing sugar
- 1 cup (250 ml) large coconut flakes, toasted (optional)

Note: If you don't have baking flour, use only 280 ml (1 cup + 2 tbsp) unbleached all-purpose flour.

Directions:

Place the rack in the bottom of the oven. Preheat the oven to 170 ° C (325 ° F).

Cake

1. In a bowl, combine the flour, icing sugar, and salt.
2. In a large, clean, fat-free bowl, whip the egg whites, cream of tartar, and vanilla with an electric mixer until soft peaks form. Gradually add granulated sugar, beating until stiff but still soft peaks form.
3. Sift the dry ingredients over the meringue, gently incorporating them as you go, folding with a whisk or spatula.
4. Pour into a non-stick, ungreased 25-cm (10-inch) pan. Bake for 45 to 50 minutes until the cake springs back after touching the surface with your finger.
5. Immediately place the pan upside down on the neck of a bottle and let the cake cool for about 3 hours or until completely cooled. Pass a thin blade of a knife between the edge of the mold and the cake, then unmold.

Icing

When ready to serve, whip cream and sugar until stiff peaks form. Garnish the top of the cake and sprinkle with coconut.

Dark Chocolate Dipped Strawberries

Preparation time: 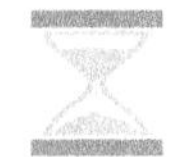

15 MINUTES

Cooking time: 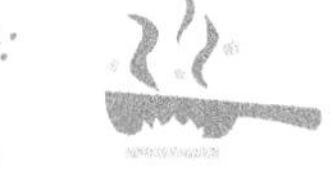

8 MINUTES

Servings: 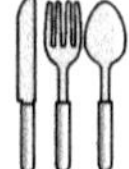

6

Here is yet another recipe that takes advantage of the tasty and nutritious value of dark chocolates. Strawberries coated with dark chocolate are a healthy and adventurous option for intermittent fasting adherents looking for a burst of fun and excitement. The recipe combines the fruity delight of strawberries with the sleek pleasure of dark chocolate melting on your tongue.

Strawberries are packed with essential vitamins such as Vitamin A, which helps to ensure optimal eyesight, and vitamin C, which aids the immune system, prevents the contraction of common diseases and improves the speed of wound healing. Strawberries are also excellent sources of fiber, which aid digestion and promote digestive system health. Strawberries also pack a punch of antioxidants, which help to reduce the effects of oxidative damage caused by free radicals within the body.

Dark chocolate, on the other hand, is also a great source of antioxidants, improves cardiac health, enhances brain function, and protects the skin from the effects of the sun's ultraviolet rays. Dark chocolate-coated strawberries can be prepared in under 10 minutes, making it a fast, convenient, and delicious dessert option.

Nutritional Information per serving:

Calories 76; Total fat: 5g; Saturated fat: 1g; Cholesterol: 1mg;
Sodium: 5mg; Carbohydrates:4g; Fiber: 1g; Sugar: 2g; Protein: 0g.

Ingredients:

- A pack of fresh strawberries
- 100g dark chocolate with 70% cocoa

Directions:

1. Melt the chocolate in a double boiler, stirring gently.

2. Prick each strawberry with a toothpick, dip two-thirds of the length of each strawberry in the chocolate.

3. Place the strawberries on a sheet of waxed paper and let cool.

Chocolate Mug Cake

Preparation time: 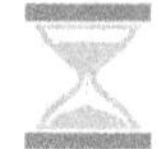
10 MINUTES

Cooking time: 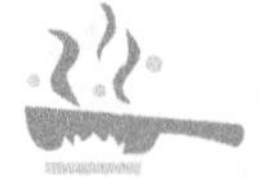
2 MINUTES

Servings: 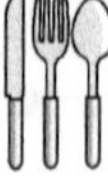
1

We all love the mug cake. With the chocolate, vanilla extract, and coconut milk? This is one tasty dessert. What more, it is low on carbs as well. One healthy sweet-tasting dish coming through!!!

Nutritional Information per serving:

Total Carbs: 30.0g; Protein: 13.4g; Fat: 24.0g; Fibre: 4.0g; Sodium: 74mg; Calories:388

Ingredients:

- ¼ cup of almond flour
- 1 large egg
- 1 tbsp. of coconut oil
- 1 tbsp. of unsweetened raw cocoa powder
- 1 tbsp. of vanilla extract
- 1 tbsp. of coconut oil
- 1 ½ tbsp. of maple syrup

Directions:

1. Get a large bowl and mix all the ingredients thoroughly until they are well combined.

2. Pour the mixture into a large mug.

3. Microwave the mixture for ninety seconds or till you confirm that it is well cooked. You can test that by dipping a toothpick in the center of the cake and check if it comes out cleanly.

4. Serve once it is done.

Peach Tart

5 HOURS

0 MINUTES

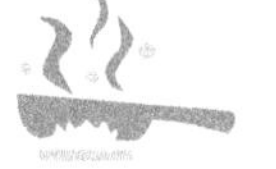

1

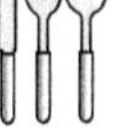

This is a delicious dessert that you are guaranteed to enjoy. An impressive mix of peaches with the tanginess of the lemon juice- your taste buds would thank you.

Nutritional Information per serving:

Total Carbs: 25.7g; Protein: 6.0g; Fat: 73.7g; Fibre: 6.8g; Sodium: 2mg; Calories:773

Ingredients:

- ¼ cup of coconut sugar
- 1 tbsp. of freshly squeezed lemon juice
- 1 prepared pie crust
- 4 cups of peeled and sliced fresh peaches

Directions:

1. Get a large bowl and mix all the ingredients together.

2. Toss and mix thoroughly.

3. Pour the mix into a pie shell. Put in the refrigerator overnight or for 5 hours before you serve.

European Hot Chocolate

<table>
<tr><td>Preparation time:
10 MINUTES</td><td>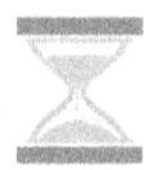</td><td>Cooking time:
5 MINUTES</td><td>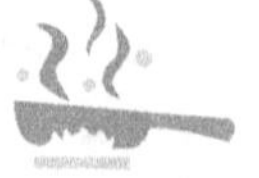</td><td>Servings:
4</td><td>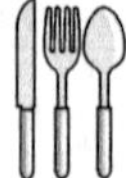</td></tr>
</table>

European hot chocolate is another fantastic exotic dessert on this list. This recipe is one of the simplest and fastest to make and offers one of the most satisfying tastes on the intermittent fasting menu. European hot chocolate can be paired with almost any dish and offers immense satisfaction to your tastebuds while enriching the body with an array of essential nutrients.

European hot chocolate has low levels of cholesterol, thereby helping to reduce the chances of high blood pressure and heart disease in the long term. Regular consumption of this dessert option can also help to lower blood sugar levels and reduce the risk of inflammation and strokes. The total preparation time is within ten minutes, and this dessert can be relished at any time of the day.

Nutritional Information per serving:

Calories 230; Total fat: 15g; Saturated fat: 1g; Cholesterol: 1mg; Sodium: 35mg; Carbohydrates: 18g; Fiber: 0g; Sugar: <1g; Protein: 4g.

Ingredients:

- 3 cups (750 mL) milk
- 1 cup (250 mL) 35% cream
- 1/4 cup (60 mL) sugar
- 1/4 cup (60 mL) cocoa
- ¼ tsp. salt
- 1 cup vanilla extract

Directions:

1. In a saucepan, simmer 2 ½ cups (625 mL) milk and 3/4 cup (180 mL) 35% cream over medium heat, stirring often.

2. Meanwhile, in a bowl, whisk together the sugar, cocoa, and salt. Whisk in the last 1/2 cup (125 mL) of cold milk and vanilla extract to form a smooth paste.

3. Reduce heat to medium-low heat and gradually add the mixture in the bowl to the milk and cream in the saucepan. Stir the entire mixture thoroughly. Heat for about 2 min or until the chocolate is steaming.

4. In a small chilled bowl, using a whisk or an electric mixer, whip the remaining cream to thicken it. Ladle the hot chocolate into four warmed cups. Spoon the whipped cream in each cup and marble the cream while stirring the spoon. Serve immediately.

Dates and Apple Bars

Preparation time: 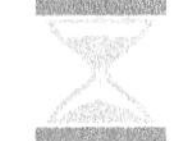	Cooking time: 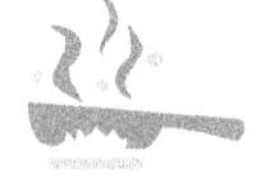	Servings: 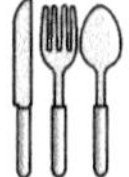
2-3 HOURS	2 MINUTES	12 BARS

Dates and apple bars are a fun, sweet, and nutritious way to treat your taste buds to an unforgettable delight. Dates and apples both contain healthy amounts of healthy sugars that make them sweet and relished by individuals of all ages. Combining these two delightful fruits into one dish simply takes the excitement to a whole new level. Dates are excellent sources of fiber, thereby promoting digestion and digestive system health. Dates are also a reliable supply of antioxidants that help to strengthen the immune system and reduce the effects of aging. Dates are also useful in helping to ease labor pains in pregnant women if eaten consistently all through the gestation period. Dates can also be used as natural sweeteners, and they have been proven to aid brain health and mental clarity.

Apples, on the other hand, are excellent for weight loss and can help to lower the risks of diabetes, heart disease, and cancers if consumed consistently over the long term. Apples also aid the maintenance of normal microbial communities within the body, thereby aiding normal body functioning. This dish is made from easy-to-source ingredients and can be ready in two hours. For your convenience, this dish can be easily refrigerated and kept for up to three days.

Nutritional Information per serving:

Calories 100; Total fat: 6g; Saturated fat: 1g; Cholesterol: 0 mg;
Sodium: 45mg; Carbohydrates: 11g; Fiber: 3g; Sugar: 6g; Protein: 2g.

Ingredients:

- 3/4 cup (180 ml) dates (preferably Medjool), pitted
- 250 ml (1 cup) dried apples, diced
- 30 ml (2 tbsp.) Chia seeds
- 15 ml (1 tbsp.) Lemon zest
- 1.25 ml (1/4 teaspoon) vanilla powder
- 1.25 ml (1/4 teaspoon) cinnamon
- 1.25 ml (1/4 tsp.) Ground ginger

Directions:

1. Rinse the dates and place them in a microwave-safe bowl. Heat the dates for 10 to 20 seconds in the microwave to soften them.

2. In the container of a food processor, mash the dates and dried apples.

3. Transfer the date mixture to a bowl. Add the chia seeds, lemon zest, vanilla, cinnamon, and ginger. Stir thoroughly until a paste is formed.

4. Line a loaf pan with parchment paper, then spread the mixture on it. Even out the surface by pressing firmly.

5. Refrigerate for 2 to 3 hours until the mixture hardens.

6. Unmold and cut into twelve bars. Keep the bars cool.

Cranberry Chutney

Preparation time:	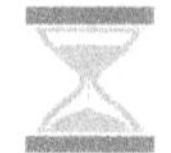	Cooking time:	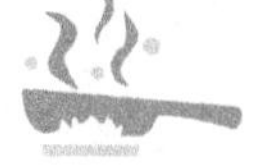	Servings:	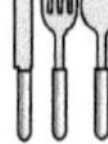
20 MINUTES		15 MINUTES		1	

The chutney is a delight to the taste buds. It is complete enough as a standalone dessert or even as a side to the mug cake we shared above for a tasty breakfast. Either way you choose to have this cranberry chutney, you would not regret it.

Nutritional Information per serving:

Total Carbs: 110.1g; Protein: 0.6g; Fat: 0.1g; Fibre: 4.9g; Sodium: 2mg; Calories:414

Ingredients:

- ¼ cup of water
- ¼ cup of fine shredded red onion
- 1 cup of coconut sugar
- 2 cups of fresh cranberries (frozen cranberries would work fine too)
- 6 whole cloves

Directions:

1. Place a small heavy bottomed saucepot on the burner on low heat.

2. Add all the ingredients into the saucepot and allow to simmer for 15 minutes.

3. Once you get a saucy consistency in the mixture, take off the heat.

4. Serve while hot.

Yogurt Parfait with Walnuts and Oatmeal

Preparation time: 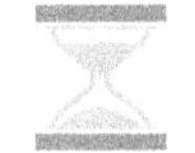

8 H TO 2 DAYS

Cooking time: 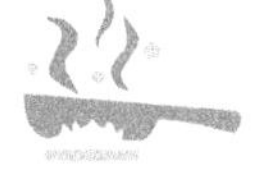

5 MINUTES

Servings: 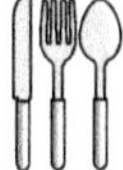

4

Yogurt parfait is a delicious, low-calorie dessert option if you are looking to switch things up a bit while eating healthy during your intermittent fasting streak. Yogurt is reputably high in protein, essential for tissue building and cellular repair. Yogurt is also made using certain lactic acid bacteria whose fermentative activities help to improve gut health and overall functioning of the digestive system. The Yogurt parfait can also help to prevent osteoporosis and ensure healthy bone density if consumed consistently. The walnuts present in the parfait ensure optimal brain health and stable moods, while the oats are rich in fiber, which also aid digestion and antioxidants that help to reverse the effects of damaging oxidative free radicals in the body.

Consuming yogurt parfait in the long-term can also help to reduce body cholesterol levels, reduce the risk of heart disease, and regulate blood sugar levels. Yogurt parfait can be cooked under 10 minutes and is prepared using ingredients that are quite easy to obtain. You can also make your yogurt parfait in advance and store it in a refrigerator for up to three days.

Nutritional Information per serving:

Calories 250; Total fat: 0.5g; Saturated fat: 0g; Cholesterol: 5mg;
Sodium: 45mg; Carbohydrates:508g; Fiber: 7g; Sugar: 39g; Protein: 14g.

Ingredients:

- 1 cup (250 mL) large oatmeal
- 1/4 cup (50 mL) chopped almonds, pecans, or walnuts (optional)
- 3 cups (750 mL) plain 2% yogurt
- 3 tbsp. (45 ml) white sugar or packed brown sugar
- 1 cup (5 ml) vanilla extract
- 2 cups (500 mL) blueberries, sliced strawberries, or raspberries

Directions:

1. In a skillet over medium heat, toast the oatmeal and walnuts while constantly stirring for 2 to 3 minutes. Immediately transfer to a bowl and let cool.

2. In a bowl, whisk the yogurt with sugar and vanilla.

3. Starting with the oat mixture, followed by the yogurt mixture and berries, divide in successive layers into four individual 1½-cup (375 mL) reusable containers with lids or in four tall glasses. Put lids or cover with plastic wrap and refrigerate for at least 8 hours, or up to two days.

Peanut Butter Cookies

30MINUTES 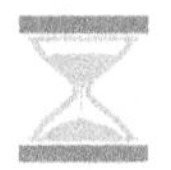

20 MINUTES 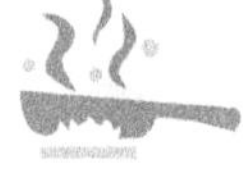

18 COOKIES 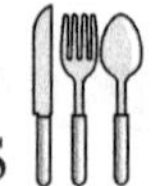

Peanut Butter cookies are an awesome dessert to have. You would probably have to prepare them beforehand so you can whip them out for a quick meal. They are prepared with natural ingredients and really easy to make.

Nutritional Information per serving:

Total Carbs: 13.2g; Protein: 3.9g; Fat: 7.8g; Fibre: 0.9g; Sodium: 47mg; Calories:136

Ingredients:

- ½ tbsp. of sea salt
- 1 cup of coconut sugar
- 1 tbsp. of pure maple syrup
- 1 cup of sugar free peanut butter
- 1 large egg
- 1 tbsp. of alcohol-free vanilla extract

Directions:

1. Heat the oven to about a temperature of 180 degrees Celsius.
2. Mix the egg, syrup, peanut butter, coconut sugar, and vanilla in a bowl. Mix thoroughly.
3. Take a tablespoon out of the dough and place it on an ungreased baking sheet. We would be making the one tablespoon per cookie spaced about 1 inch apart on the baking sheet.
4. Press down the dough with the fork, then use the same fork to form a crosshatch pattern on the dough. Sprinkle salt lightly on the cookies.
5. Bake the dough for 5 minutes at 160 degrees Celsius, then turn the baking sheet and bake for another 5 minutes.
6. Once the cookies are golden brown on the edges, it means they are done.
7. Take out the cookies and allow them to cool down for about 10 minutes before you serve.

Pumpkin Pie with Greek Yogurt

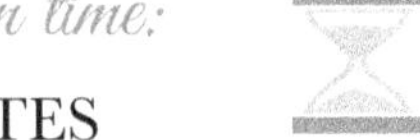

55 MINUTES

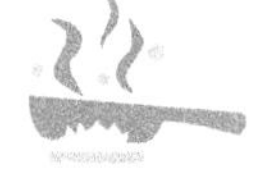

45 MINUTES

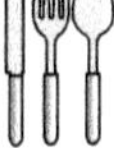

8

Pumpkin pie is another classic American favorite whose nutritional benefits and unbeatable taste make it an integral component of the intermittent fasting recipe list. Pumpkin pie is rich in Vitamin A, which aids optimal eyesight and enhances immune system activity. Pumpkin pie is also rich in potassium, which aids clotting of blood and enhances nervous system function; vitamin C, which aids speedy healing of wounds; and iron, which enhances the synthesis of red blood cells.

Greek yogurt, on the other hand, adds a burst of protein to this dish for tissue building and cellular repair while also helping with weight loss and the prevention of cardiac diseases. Pumpkin pie with Greek Yogurt can be made from scratch for under one hour and can be kept refrigerated for up to two days.

Nutritional Information per serving:

Calories 170; Total fat: 5g; Saturated fat: 0g; Cholesterol: 0 mg; Sodium: 70 mg; Carbohydrates:16g; Fiber: 3g; Sugar: 10g; Protein: 17g.

Ingredients:

Crust

- 175 g (1 ¼ cup) unbleached all-purpose flour
- 30 ml (2 tbsp.) Sugar
- 1 ml (¼ teaspoon) salt
- 115 g (½ cup) cold unsalted butter, diced
- 60 ml (¼ cup) plain 2% yogurt

Garnish

- 5 ml (1 tsp.) Corn starch
- 2.5 ml (½ teaspoon) ground cinnamon
- 1 ml (¼ teaspoon) ground nutmeg
- Two eggs
- 1 ½ cups (375 ml) store-bought plain pumpkin puree
- One can of 300 ml sweetened condensed milk
- 125 ml (½ cup) 35% cream
- 30 ml (2 tbsp.) Icing sugar

Directions:

Crust

1. In a food processor, combine the flour, sugar, and salt. Add the butter and stir a few seconds at a time until an even consistency is achieved.
2. Add the yogurt and mix again until the dough just begins to form. Remove the dough from the food processor and use it to form a disc with your hands.
3. Cover with plastic wrap and refrigerate for 30 minutes.
4. Place the rack in the bottom of the oven and preheat the oven to 190 ° C (375 ° F).
5. On a lightly floured work surface, roll out the dough and line a 23 cm (9 in) diameter pie plate. Cut off excess dough 1 cm (½ inch) outside of the pan. Fold the dough to form a double layer.
6. Scallop the border (with your fingers, form a series of curves to decorate it). Reserve.

Garnish

1. In a bowl, combine the corn starch and spices. Using a whisk, add the eggs. Add the pumpkin puree and sweetened condensed milk. Mix until well combined and pour into crust.
2. Bake for 35 to 40 minutes or until the filling is slightly wiggly in the center. Let cool on the rack.
3. In a bowl, whip the cream with the sugar until stiff peaks form. Using a pastry bag fitted with a fluted nozzle, decorate the edge of the pie or garnish the wedges when ready to serve.

Raspberry Jam with Lemon and Chia seed

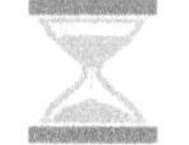

Preparation time:
3 H 20 MINUTES

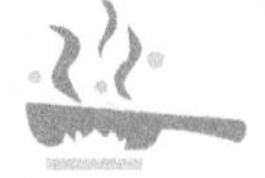

Cooking time:
20 MINUTES

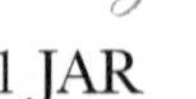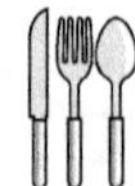

Servings:
1 JAR

The Raspberry jam is a wonderful addition to any of your desserts. It is an awesome sugar-free Jam recipe with a sweet, delicious taste. You can add this to your yogurt or cookies and scones. You can store this jam frozen for up to 2 months.

Nutritional Information per serving:

Total Carbs: 7.5g; Protein: 0.5g; Fat: 0.5g; Fibre: 1.9g; Sodium: 1mg; Calories:34

Ingredients:

- ½ pint of fresh raspberries
- 1 tbsp. of chia seeds
- 1 tbsp. of freshly squeezed lemon juice
- 1 tbsp. of lemon zest
- 2 ½ tbsp. of pure maple syrup

Directions:

1. Get a saucepan going over a burner on medium high heat. Add the Lemon juice, maple syrup, raspberries, and lemon zest. Cover simmer and stir occasionally. Cook for like 10 minutes.

2. Once the mixture begins to thicken, remove the cover from the saucepan. Set the burner to high heat and boil the mixture while stirring often. Continue cooking till it starts looking and thickening like a sauce.

3. Pour in the chia seeds and stir. Cook again – without covering the saucepan- for another 2 minutes, then take off the heat.

4. Allow it to cool. Transfer the cooled Jam into an airtight container and refrigerate. The thickness of the jam would increase with an increase in refrigeration. Allow a minimum of 3 hours to refrigerate before use.

500 Calorie Meals for Women

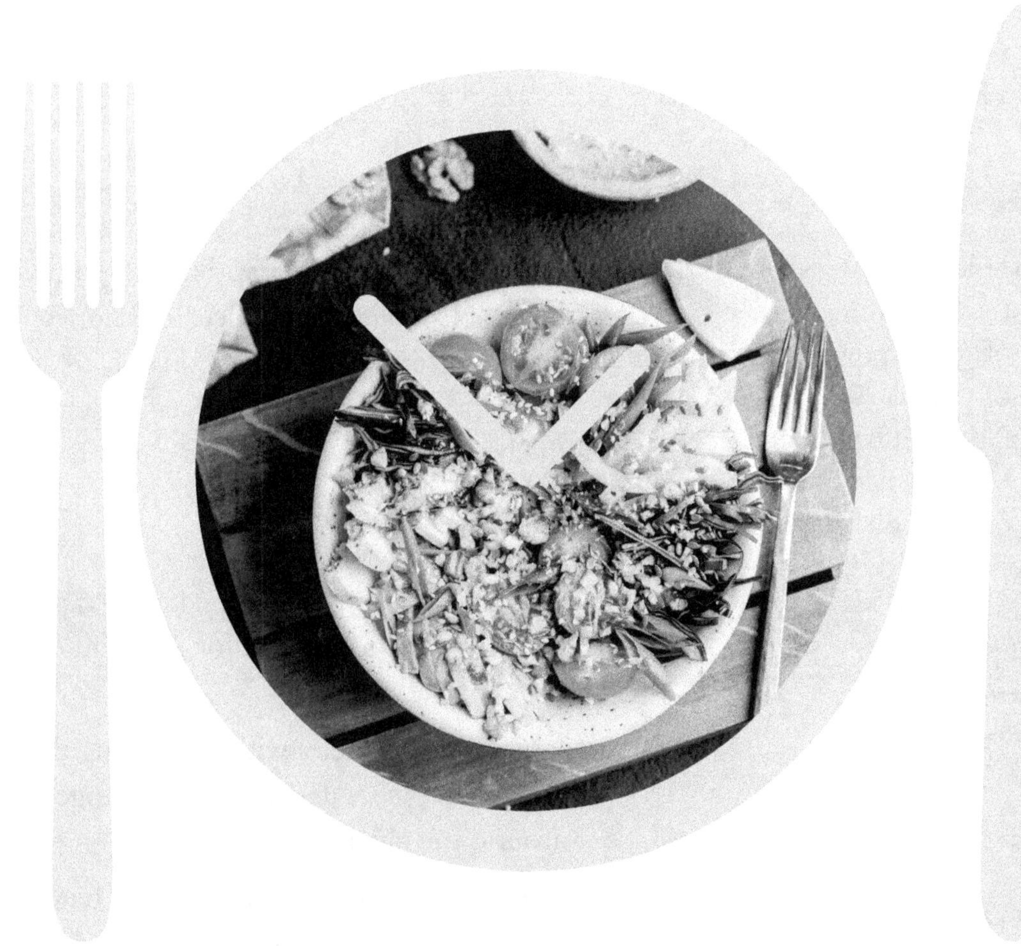

Cajun Grilled Chicken

Preparation time: 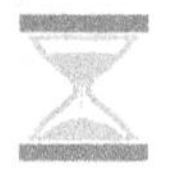

14 HOURS

Cooking time: 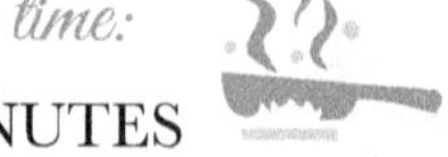

1 H 20 MINUTES

Servings: 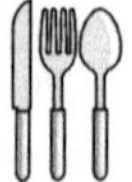

4

Cajun grilled chicken brings another dimension to exactly how delicious chicken can truly be. Cajun chicken utilizes a series of exotic spices to make a nutritious and exceptionally-tasting grilled chicken. Cajun grilled chicken has a high protein content, which aids in building muscle and repairing worn-out cells. This dish also has a high calcium content, thereby helping to build strong teeth and bones while reducing the risks of hemorrhage on sustaining physical trauma. Cajun grilled chicken promotes optimal cardiac health, reduces the risk of cancers, and is low in calories, thereby aiding weight loss.
Cajun grilled chicken can be cooked under two hours, requires relatively common equipment, and can be enjoyed at any time of the day. This dish can also be preserved in the refrigerator for up to three days.

Nutritional Information per serving:

Calories 520; Total fat: 23g; Saturated fat: 3.5g; Cholesterol: 80mg; Sodium: 150mg; Carbohydrates: 42g; Fiber: 16g; Sugar: 10g; Protein: 45g

Ingredients:

- One whole chicken
- 2 tsp of salt
- 1 tbsp of garlic powder
- 2 tbsp of paprika
- 1 tsp of Espelette pepper
- 1 tbsp of Provence herbs
- 4 tbsp of olive oil
- One lemon (juiced)
- 1 tbsp of honey
- ½ pumpkin
- Two large carrots
- 400g sweet potatoes

Directions:

1. Combine salt, garlic, paprika, chili, Provence herbs, olive oil, lemon juice, and honey in a large freezer bag. Shake vigorously to combine the ingredients, and then place the chicken in the bag and seal to allow the chicken to soak in the marinade. Leave in the refrigerator for 12 hours.

2. Take the chicken out of the bag and place it in a dish. Bake the chicken for 20 minutes at 190 ° C.

3. Wash the vegetables without peeling them. Cut them into pieces if necessary. Arrange them around the chicken.

4. Add 4 tbsp of water to the freezer bag, shake and pour over the vegetables.

5. Cook the chicken over medium heat for 1 hour.

6. Serve hot and enjoy.

Salmon Fillet with Fresh Spinach

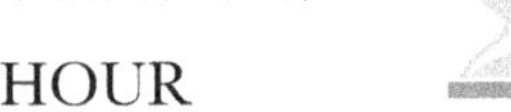

Preparation time: 1 HOUR

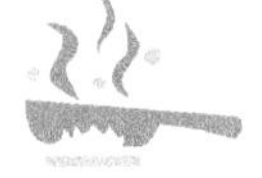

Cooking time: 40 MINUTES

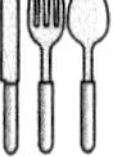

Servings: 4

A delicious, exquisite taste, ease of preparation, and an array of essential nutrients are the key hallmarks of the Salmon fillet and fresh spinach dish. Salmon is rich in antioxidants that help to reduce oxidative damage by free radicals. Salon also contains a plethora of vitamins and minerals, most notably Vitamin B12, potassium, and selenium, which all play key roles in disease prevention and strengthening the immune system. Salmon is also a rich source of Omega-3 fatty acids, which aid in weight loss, prevention of heart disease, and optimal brain health.

Spinach, on the other hand, is also a rich source of vitamins, with high concentrations of Vitamin C, which strengthens the immune system and accelerates wound healing, and Vitamin A, which enhances excellent eyesight. Spinach is also an abundant source of iron, which helps to prevent anemia.

Nutritional Information per serving:

Calories 500; Total fat: 28g; Saturated fat: 7 g; Cholesterol: 85 mg; Sodium: 370 mg; Carbohydrates: 22g; Fiber: 2g; Sugar: 6g; Protein: 37g

Ingredients:

- 800g Salmon fillet
- One lemon
- One leek (small)
- Two medium carrots
- 2 tbsp. olive oil
- 1 tsp. salt
- Three handfuls of fresh Spinach
- Two balls of mozzarella
- 2 tbsp. "pure butter" puff pastry
- One egg
- 10cl milk

Directions:

1. In a pan with two tablespoons of olive oil, heat a handful of leeks and carrots cut into pieces and add salt and pepper. Let the preparation cool completely.
2. Heat a small saucepan of hot water, and add in a pinch of salt. Add two handfuls of Spinach to the hot water and leave for 5 seconds. Drain the Spinach immediately and let them cool on a clean cloth.
3. Roll out the first puff pastry and place it in a pie pan for evenness while leaving the baking paper underneath. Add the bits of fried vegetables to the puff pastry, and place the fish on top. Season the mixture with salt and add the whole lemon zest and the chopped mozzarella.
4. Arrange the spinach leaf by leaf over the salmon. Remove the stems as you go. Cover with the second puff pastry and roll up the edges and preheat the oven to 180 degrees.
5. Brush the top of the puff pastry with a little milk and the egg. Leave the preparation in the fridge until you're ready to bake. Cover with baking paper and cook for 40 minutes.
6. Serve hot with a salad of fresh spinach and tomatoes, and lemon wedges. Accompany the salad with a vinaigrette.

Farro Salad

 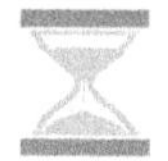
35 MINUTES

 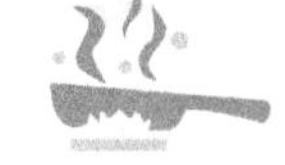
25 MINUTES

 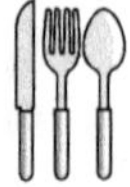
4

Farro salad is a simple and tasty dish rich in fibers and filled with a wide array of antioxidants that help to reverse the unhealthy effects of free radicals in the body. Farro salad is also a rich source of protein, and its low-calorie content makes it helpful in shedding excess fat.

Farro salad can be prepared in one hour and can be left for two days in a refrigerator.

Nutritional Information per serving:

Calories 500; Total fat: 19g; Saturated fat: 5g; Cholesterol: 10mg; Sodium: 590mg; Carbohydrates: 69g; Fiber: 8g; Sugar: 3g; Protein: 20g.

Ingredients:

Salad

- 2 cups of vegetable broth
- 1 cup of farro (or barley)
- 1 Lebanese cucumber
- 1/2 red onion
- 1/2 cup cherry tomatoes
- 1/4 cup flat-leaf parsley
- 1/4 cup green olives or Kalamata
- Four organic Medjool dates
- 4-5 branches of kale

Mediterranean Chia Dressing

- 3 tbsp. tablespoon olive oil
- 1 C. 1/4 teaspoon PRANA organic whole ProactivChia seeds
- 1 C. tablespoon of apple cider vinegar
- One garlic clove, grated
- One pinch of dried oregano
- sea salt and freshly ground pepper, to taste

Directions:

The salad

1. Rinse the farro thoroughly, then drain it. In a saucepan, combine the farro and vegetable broth, and bring to a boil. Reduce heat to low, cover, and cook for 25 minutes or until the grains are tender to the taste. If any broth remains at the bottom of the pot, drain the grains.

2. Meanwhile, cut the cucumber into slices and then the slices in halves. Finely chop the red onion, cut the tomatoes in half, roughly chop the parsley, pit the dates and thinly slice them, and finely chop the kale.

3. Prepare the vinaigrette.

4. In a large bowl, combine farro with remaining ingredients and dressing, and toss. Add the salt and pepper.

Mediterranean chia dressing

Put all the vinaigrette ingredients in a mason jar, stir vigorously, and set aside.

Mexican Burritos with Rice, Red Beans with Tomato & Cheese

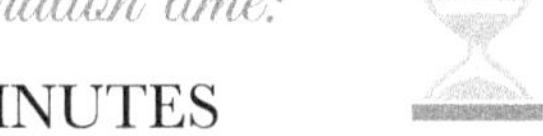

Preparation time:

25 MINUTES

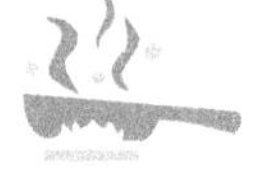

Cooking time:

15 MINUTES

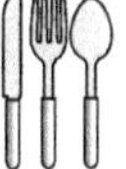

Servings:

6

Mexican burritos are a fantastic source of a wide variety of food nutrients. Add the nutritive value of this delicacy to its impeccable taste, and you would understand why Mexican burritos have such an incredible reputation. The Mexican burrito aids the proper functioning of the immune system, enhances weight loss, and supplies the body with proteins needed for muscle building and tissue repair. Mexican burritos are also rich in Vitamins B, C, D, and E, which prevent a plethora of diseases, aid the immune system, enhance bone strength, and even boost fertility.

Nutritional Information per serving:

Calories 480; Total fat: 16g; Saturated fat: 4.5g; Cholesterol: 5mg; Sodium: 940mg; Carbohydrates: 72g; Fiber: 10g; Sugar: 11g; Protein: 17g.

Ingredients:

- Six large wheat wraps or tortillas
- One small can of red kidney beans, drained (250 g)
- 190g cooked tomato sauce (190 g)
- 200g grated cheddar cheese
- Two tablespoons chopped cilantro (frozen)
- One teaspoon of cumin
- Two tablespoons of sriracha chili sauce (Asian grocery store)
- 100g long-grain rice
- Six tablespoons of sour cream

Directions:

1. Cook the rice in a large pot of salted boiling water. Drain.

2. In a large bowl or salad bowl, combine the beans, tomato sauce, chili sauce, cilantro, and cumin.

3. Spread each wrap of tortilla with a tablespoon of crème Fraiche. Arrange the fillings in a horizontal strip: 1/6 of the rice, 1/6 of the beans, and 1/6 of the cheese. Fold the left and right sides over the stuffing, then fold the bottom of the wrap over the stuffing and roll it up.

4. Heat for 30 seconds to 1 minute in the microwave.

5. Serve immediately.

Italian Pasta and Beans

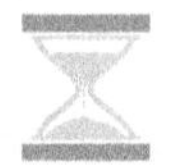

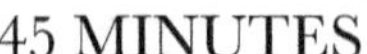
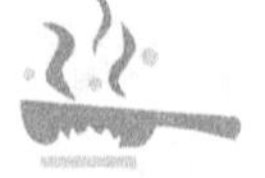

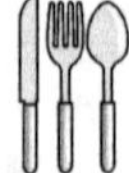

The Italian pasta and beans dish is a perfect combination for energy, low calories, and bodybuilding proteins. This dish contains just enough sodium for optimal nervous system function and is completely free of cholesterol. Pasta is also a great source of folic acid, which greatly aids fetal development. Beans are also rich sources of antioxidants that control the effects of oxidative free radicals that cause premature aging. Consuming Italian pasta and beans regularly has been proven to reduce the risks of cancer and diabetes while encouraging a healthy appetite.

Nutritional Information per serving:

Calories 470; Total fat: 25g; Saturated fat: 2.5g; Cholesterol: 0mg; Sodium: 900mg; Carbohydrates: 70g; Fiber: 7g; Sugar: 4g; Protein: 17g.

Ingredients:

- 250g cooked white beans, drained
- 200g of dry pasta (for example, the one usually used for minestrones)
- 400g tomato pulp
- One large carrot
- One stalk of celery
- ½ liter of vegetable broth
- One onion
- Two cloves garlic
- One bay leaf
- One branch of sage
- One sprig of thyme
- 3 tbsp of olive oil
- A little Parmesan to serve (or malted yeast for a 100% vegetable version)

Directions:

1. Peel and mince the onion. Peel and crush the garlic. Peel the carrot. Cut the celery stalk and the carrot into small cubes (about 5mm per side).

2. Heat the oil in an oven. Add the onion, garlic, and diced carrots, and celery, then the herbs.

3. Sauté the entire mixture over low heat and covered for 5 minutes, then add the tomato pulp and broth. Cook the preparation over low heat for 30 minutes.

4. Meanwhile, take about 1/3 of the beans and mash them with a fork or with a hand-held potato masher.

5. Bring water to the boil for the pasta.

6. Add the whole and mashed beans with the tomato vegetables and cook for about 10 minutes.

7. Cook the pasta according to the package directions and drain when it is cooked to your liking.

8. Add the beans and tomato mixture to the pasta and serve immediately with grated Parmesan cheese.

600 Calorie Meals for Women

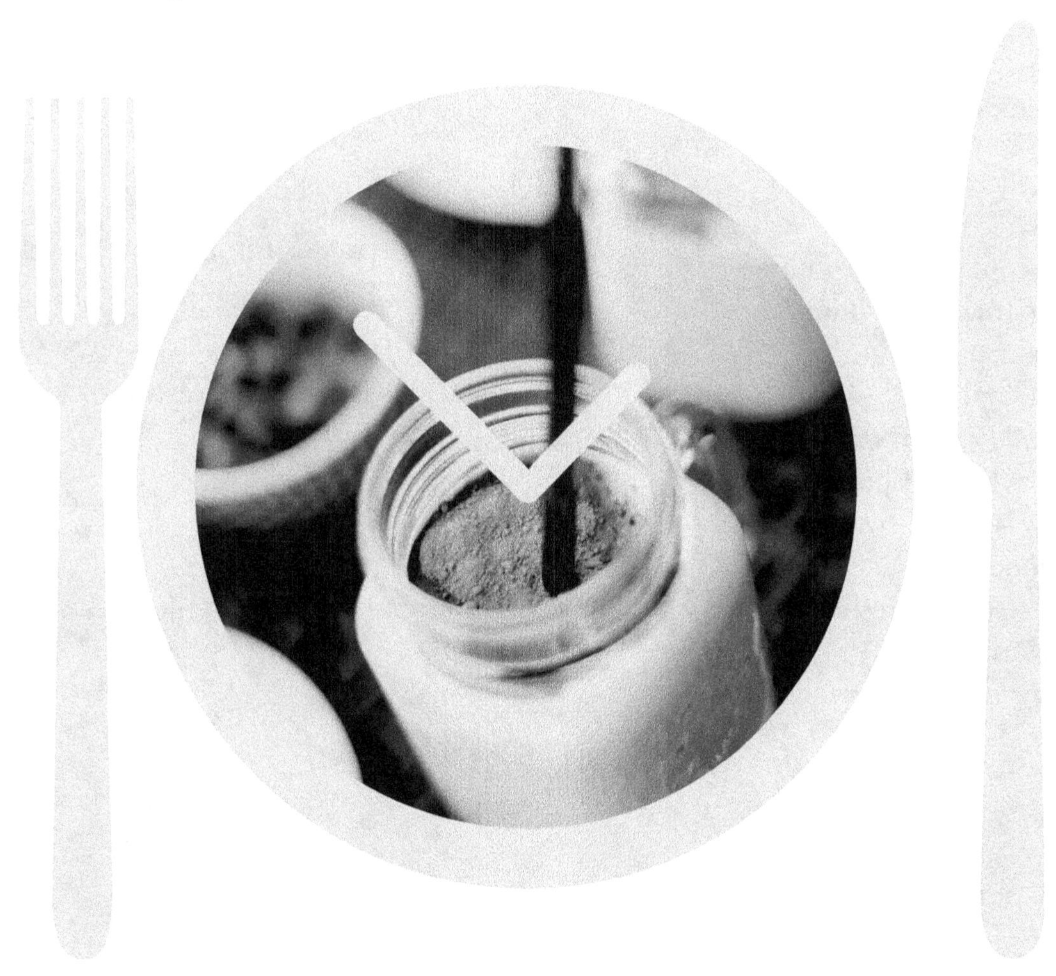

Veggie Sandwich with Hummus

Preparation time:
10 MINUTES 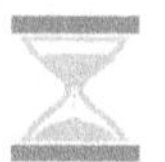

Cooking time:
5 MINUTES 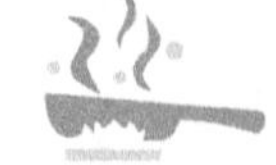

Servings:
6 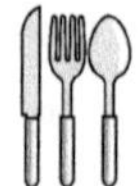

This unique dish combines hummus with a collection of nutritious vegetables, including Spinach and brussels sprouts, while incorporating the goodness of avocados and mozzarella cheese. This veggie sandwich is packed with protein for tissue building and cellular repair and fiber that ensures smooth digestion and ensures exceptional gut health. This sandwich also has a low glycemic index, thereby helping to control blood sugar levels.

Nutritional Information per serving:

Calories 590; Total fat: 37g; Saturated fat: 7g; Cholesterol: 60mg; Sodium: 610mg; Carbohydrates: 61g; Fiber: 18g; Sugar: 6g; Protein: 17g.

Ingredients:

- Four slices of wholemeal bread
- One container of Fontaine Santé traditional hummus
- 2 cups Spinach
- ½ cucumber,
- 125 ml (½ cup) sprouts
- One avocado ripe, sliced
- A few slices of sweet pickles (optional)
- One scoop of fresh mozzarella
- ½ tsp. salt
- ¼ tsp. fresh pepper

Directions:

1. Lightly toast the slices of bread.
2. Generously spread hummus over each slice, add a layer of green veggies, cucumber slices, sprouts, avocado slices, a few slices of sweet pickles if desired, fresh mozzarella, salt, and pepper.
3. Add cucumber slices and some more veggies.
4. Close the sandwich and enjoy.

Whole Grain Linguine Pasta with Clams

Preparation time:
25 MINUTES

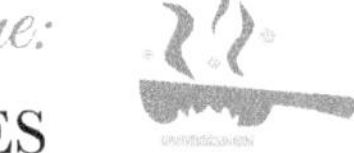

Cooking time:
20 MINUTES

Servings:
4

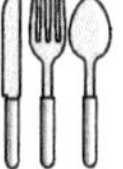

Linguine pasta with clams and tomatoes is an excellent low-calorie energy source that allows you to derive the healthy carbohydrates you require to function optimally while preventing unhealthy weight gain. This dish is also low in sodium and cholesterol but is rich in folic acid. Through the clams, this dish is enriched with omega-3 fatty acids, which help to reduce the risk of cardiac complications and improve mental health.

Nutritional Information per serving:

Calories 580; Total fat: 14 g; Saturated fat: 3 g; Cholesterol: 80 mg; Sodium: 240 mg; Carbohydrates: 68 g; Fiber: 1g; Sugar: 3 g; Protein: 50g.

Ingredients:

- 350g Linguine pasta
- 1kg Clams
- 100g Sun-dried tomatoes
- Two garlic cloves
- 5cl Dry white wine
- 5cl olive oil
- Salt
- Pepper

Directions:

1. Rinse the clams thoroughly to remove the sand.

2. Cut the sun-dried tomatoes into strips.

3. In a large skillet, heat three tablespoonfuls of oil. Add the clams, the sundried tomatoes, and sprinkle the chopped garlic, salt, and pepper. Sauté for 10 minutes, stirring often, then pour in the white wine.

4. At the same time, cook the pasta in boiling salted water according to the package directions (about 8 min.) Drain, season with olive oil, and pour into a dish previously heated.

5. Add the clams to the tomatoes, mix gently and serve immediately.

6. Serve with a bit of grated Parmesan cheese.

Bean and Turkey Slow Cooker Chili

 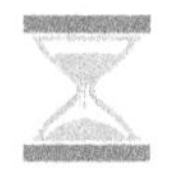
4-8 HOURS

 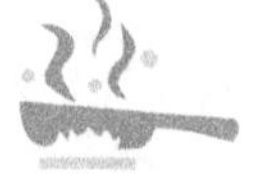
4-8 HOURS

 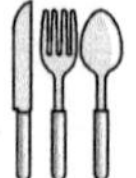
8

This dish provides a wide variety of essential nutrients, and the fact that it tastes absolutely fascinating is a great plus. Turkey is a rich source of protein, which is needed for bodybuilding and cellular repair. Turkey is also an abundant source of zinc, a macronutrient that helps to strengthen the immune system. Beans are rich in proteins and folate; they contain antioxidants that prevent oxidative damage by free radicals, improve heart health, and help to reduce the risks of cancer. This dish can be made within 4 hours and 15 minutes of preparation.

Nutritional Information per serving:

Calories 630; Total fat: 7g; Saturated fat: 1 g; Cholesterol: 70 mg; Sodium: 740 mg; Carbohydrates: 84g; Fiber: 12 g; Sugar: 15g; Protein: 60g.

Ingredients:

- 2 tbsp. vegetable oil
- 1 lb. ground turkey
- Two cans (284 mL) condensed tomato soup
- Two cans (540 mL) kidney beans, drained
- One can (540 mL) black beans, drained
- ½ medium onion, chopped
- 2 tbsp. chili powder
- 1 tbsp. red pepper flakes
- 1/2 tsp. garlic powder
- 1/2 tsp. cumin
- One pinch of pepper
- One pinch of allspice (allspice)
- ½ tsp. salt

Directions:

1. Heat the oil in a skillet over medium heat. Sauté meat until browned. Drain.

2. Oil the inside of a slow cooker container and add the turkey, tomato soup, beans, and onion. Season with chili powder, chili flakes, garlic powder, cumin, pepper, allspice, and salt.

3. Cover and cook on low power for 8 hours or on high power for 4 hours.

Banana Chocolate Protein Smoothie

Preparation time:	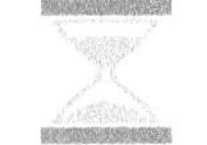	Cooking time:	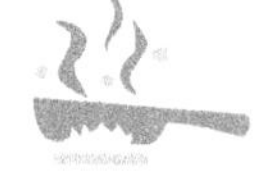	Servings:	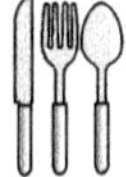
10 MINUTES		0 MINUTES		4	

The banana chocolate protein smoothie is a simple and nutritious ensemble that integrates the distinctive taste of chocolates with the unbeatable health benefits of bananas. The smoothie is low in calories and therefore encourages weight loss. The high fiber content aids ease of digestion and the bananas contain an array of powerful antioxidants that counteract the damaging effects of free radicals. The smoothie may also help to lower blood pressure, thereby improving long-term cardiac health, and also improve brain function.

The smoothie is easy to put together, can be prepared under ten minutes, and can be refrigerated for up to a day.

Nutritional Information per serving:

Calories 600; Total fat: 19g; Saturated fat: 2g; Cholesterol: 0 mg; Sodium: 780mg; Carbohydrates: 48g; Fiber: 8g; Sugar: 20g; Protein: 61g.

Ingredients:

- One frozen banana
- 25g cocoa powder without sugar
- 1 tbsp. peanut butter
- 200 ml higher protein soy milk
- 1 tbsp. chia seeds
- 2 tbsp. oat bran

Directions:

1. Place the banana, chia seeds, part of the vegetable milk of your choice (to be able to adjust the texture later), and the oatmeal in a blender.

2. Mix for the first time. Now add the peanut butter or other oilseeds (almonds, cashews, etc.)

3. Blend a second time. Gradually add the rest of the vegetable milk until you get the desired texture.

4. Serve and enjoy.

Sides

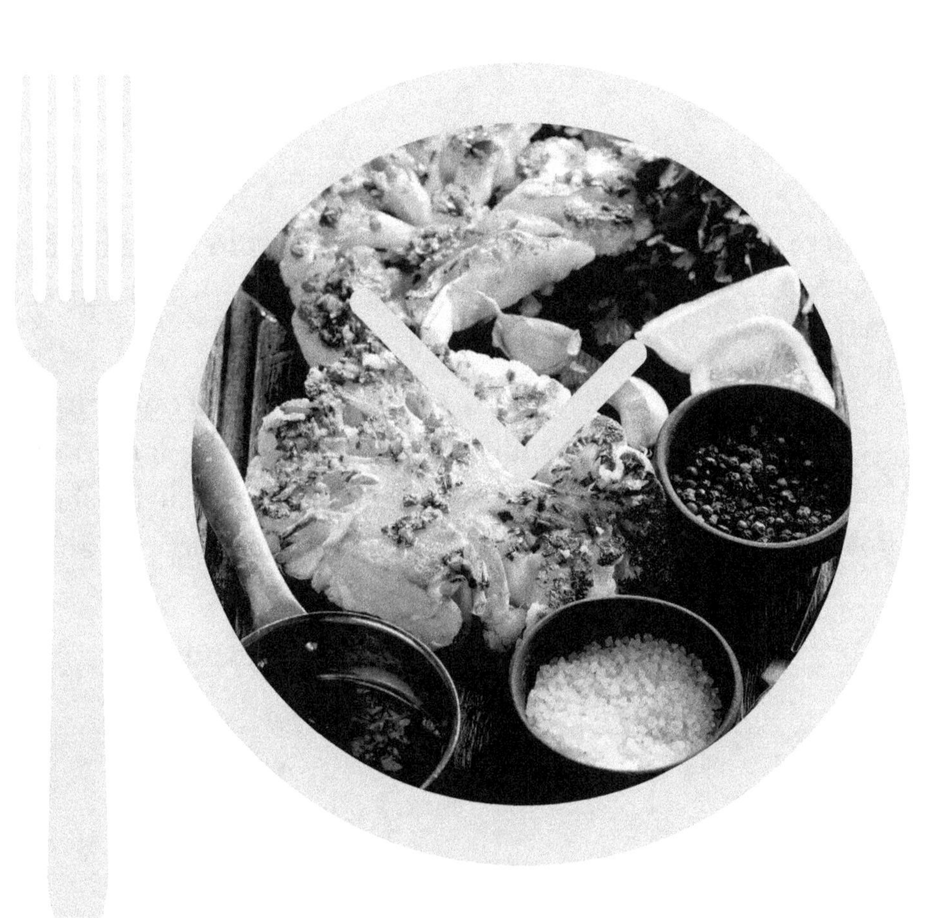

Chili-Roasted Cauliflower Steaks

Preparation time: 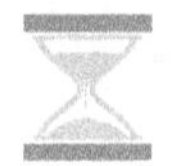
35 MINUTES

Cooking time: 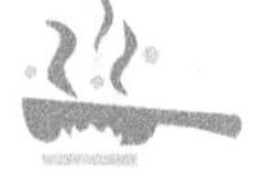
30 MINUTES

Servings: 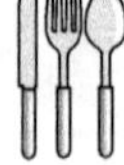
4

It is amazing that just a pinch of chili flakes can help to boost the body's metabolism and mood, making it a good meal for women over fifty. With the presence of cauliflower, this is one delicious meal that you cannot afford to miss.

Nutritional Information per serving:

In one serving, you get 2.8 g of protein, 7.2 g of fat, 4.4 g of Net Carbs, 335 mg of Sodium, 442 mg of Potassium, and 97 Calories.

Ingredients:

- 1 medium cauliflower cut into six steak-like pieces
- ½ tbsp. of fine salt
- ¼ tbsp. of crushed red pepper flakes
- 2 tbsp. pf extra virgin olive oil
- Black pepper, freshly grounded

Directions:

1. Use parchment paper to line a baking tray. Next, preheat the oven to 400 degrees Fahrenheit.
2. Drizzle a tbsp. of olive oil on each of the cauliflower pieces, making sure to rub the oil all over them. Next, sprinkle crushed pepper flakes, freshly grounded pepper, and salt evenly on the pieces.
3. Bake for thirty minutes and serve.

Ras el Hanout Roasted Red Cabbage

Preparation time:	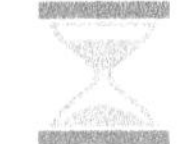	Cooking time:	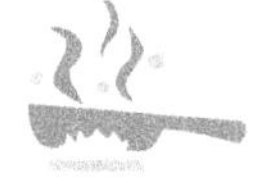	Servings:	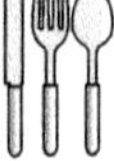
1 H 20 MINUTES		1 H 10 MINUTES		6	

This is one cabbage that gets people as excited as when they eat bacon. It is a nice side meal to throw in on some lunch when cabbage makes it to your craving. Let's learn to make it then.

Nutritional Information per serving:

In one serving, you get 1 g of protein, 4.6 g of Fat, 2.6 g of Net Carbs, 338 mg of Sodium, 132 mg of Potassium, and 60 Calories.

Ingredients:

- ½ tbsp. of extra virgin olive oil
- ½ tbsp. of ras el hanout spice blend
- 1 pound of red/green cabbage
- 1 tbsp. of Himalayan salt

Directions:

1. Use parchment paper to line a baking tray and preheat the oven to 350 degrees Fahrenheit
2. Cut the cabbage into 1-inch-thick wedges and lay them on the baking tray.
3. Drizzle the cabbage wedges with olive oil and sprinkle salt and ras el hanout blend on them. Toss lightly and rub to ensure that the wedges are well coated with seasoning and oil.
4. Bake for thirty minutes until the cabbage wedges become nicely golden brown. Remove the tray and cover it with foil. Bake for another thirty minutes. It will steam and become tender in the foil-covered tray.
5. Serve after and enjoy.

Meals for Breakfast, Lunch and Dinner

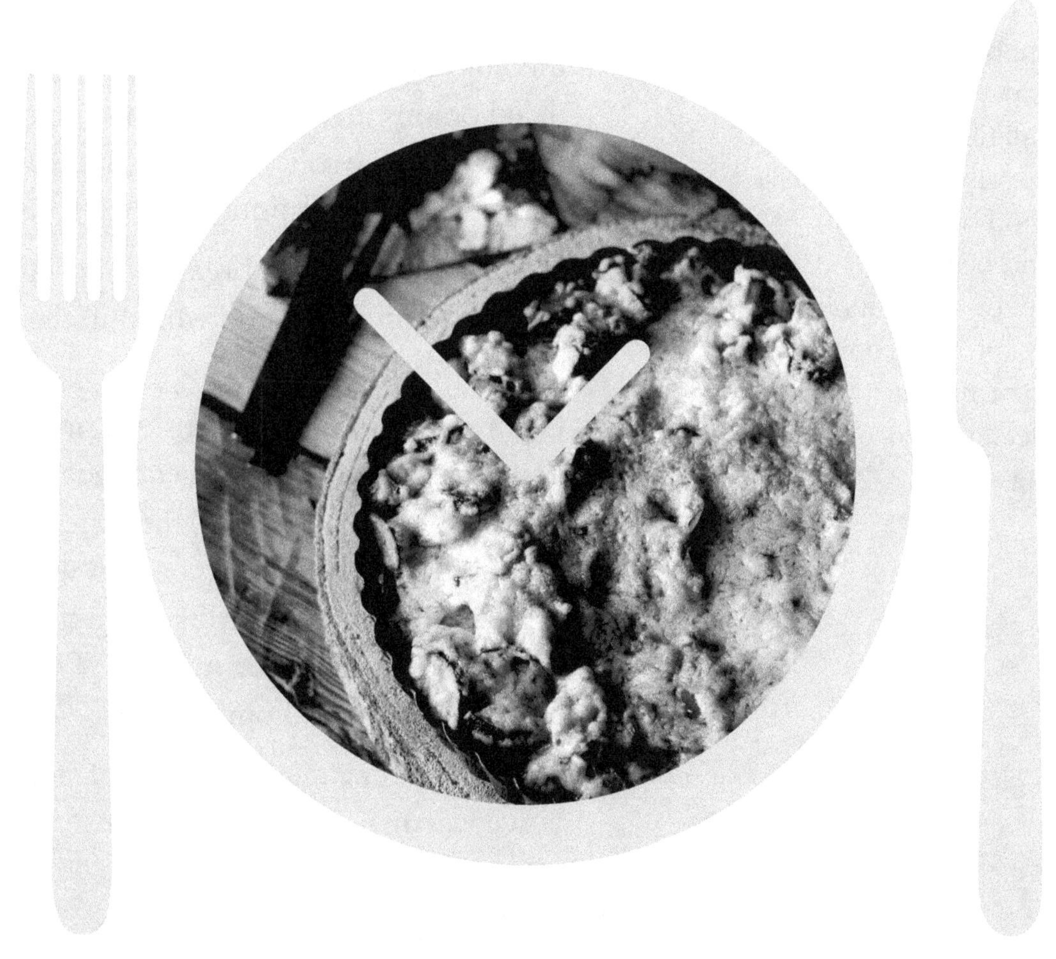

Casserole

Preparation time: 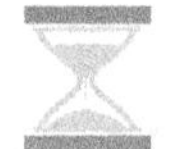
10 H 25 MINUTES

Cooking time: 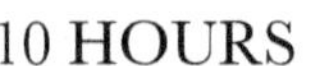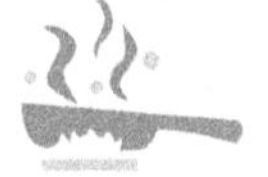
10 HOURS

Servings: 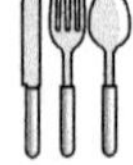
2

This is an ideal breakfast dish that should be prepared in advance. You can prepare this dish by two days or even a day before you eat it. This only ensures that you have the meal readily available and saves you the hassle of preparing a breakfast dish well into the afternoon.

Nutritional Information per serving:

Total Carbs: 11.4g; Protein: 41.3g; Fat: 37.4g; Fibre: 1.6g; Sodium: 288mg; Calories:581

Ingredients:

- 1 small seeded, peeled, and sliced butternut squash
- 1 tbsp. of freshly grounded black pepper
- 1 small diced yellow onion
- 1 tbsp. of red pepper flakes
- 1 pound of 85% lean ground beef
- 1 tbsp. of coconut oil
- 1 tbsp. of garlic powder
- 1 cup of full fat unsweetened coconut milk
- 12 eggs

Directions:

1. Start by cooking the 1-pound ground beef in a skillet placed over a burner on medium heat. Then add the spices and diced onions into the skillet and cook till the onions become soft. This would ideally take between 10 to 12 minutes.

2. Get a large bowl and break in the eggs. Then add milk to it and whisk till they are thoroughly mixed.

3. Get a slow cooker. 6-quart sized preferably and grease the inside with coconut oil. Add the butternut squash in it, then the cooked ground beef. Then cover it all up with the egg and milk mixture. Make sure the beef is totally immersed in the mixture. Then cook on low heat for 10 hours.

4. Once it is done, take out the beef and slice. Serve warm.

Chia Bowl

Preparation time: 

30 MINUTES

Cooking time: 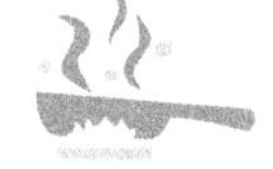

25 MINUTES

Servings: 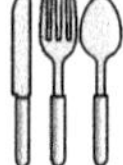

1

The leaves are down, the breeze blows gently in the morning, and that Autumn feeling creeps in. This breakfast would take you back to mornings like these. With an accompanying flavor of cinnamon and cranberry, you can have this breakfast no matter what season we are in.

Nutritional Information per serving:

Total Carbs: 67.2g; Protein: 17.8g; Fat: 15.6g; Fibre: 16.8g; Sodium: 352mg; Calories:471

Ingredients:

- ¼ tbsp. of salt
- ½ tbsp. of ground cinnamon
- ½ cup of unsweetened almond milk
- 1 tbsp. of dried sugar free cranberries
- 1 cup of gluten-free oats
- 1 tbsp. of cut almonds
- 1 tbsp. of halved macadamia nuts
- 3 tbsp. of chia seeds
- 3 cups of cold water

Directions:

1. Boil water and salt in a saucepan on high heat. Once the water starts to boil, add the oats and leave for a minute.

2. Reduce the heat from the burner to medium low. Then add the almond milk and stir.

3. Add the cinnamon, chia seeds, cut macadamia nuts, diced almonds, and the dried cranberries, then stir.

4. Allow everything to cook for about 20 minutes, still on medium low heat while you keep stirring it occasionally. Continue to do this until the chia seeds are like gel and have turned soft.

5. Turn off the heat and serve as is.

Hash Brown Bake with Turkey and Egg White

Preparation time: 
1 H 15 MINUTES

Cooking time: 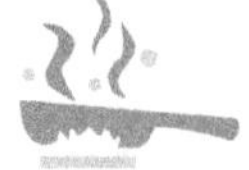
45 MINUTES

Servings: 
16

Breakfast, healthy, tasty, with a feel of exuberance, this is the dish for you. So easy to prepare, so tasty to the buds, and packed with nutrients, this meal is the ideal breakfast dish or even for any time of the day.

Nutritional Information per serving:

Total Carbs: 5.1g; Protein: 10.7g; Fat: 7.4g; Fibre: 0.5g; Sodium: 344mg; Calories:137

Ingredients:

- ½ tbsp. of grounded cayenne pepper
- 1 pound of shredded russet potatoes
- 1 tbsp. of olive oil
- 1 pound of 85% lean ground turkey
- 1 ½ tbsp. of salt
- 1 ½ tbsp. of fresh grounded black pepper
- 12 large eggs

Directions:

1. Heat the oven to a temperature of 190 degrees Celsius.

2. Get a casserole dish and grease it with cooking spray, and set it aside.

3. Get a medium sized skillet on the burner. Over medium heat, pour the olive oil in the skillet and add the ground turkey. Cook in the skillet for about 6 minutes till the turkey is no longer pink colored.

4. Once the turkey is done cooking, pour it into a large bowl. Add all the other ingredients to it and mix thoroughly.

5. Then pure the mixture into the baking dish that has been prepared. Bake the mixture for about 40 minutes till the top is solid. You can as well dip a toothpick in it to check. If the toothpick comes out clean, then it means the bake is done.

6. Take out of the oven and allow it to cool down for about 30 minutes.

7. Cut the bake into 16 pieces and serve.

Cran-Orange Oatmeal

20 MINUTES

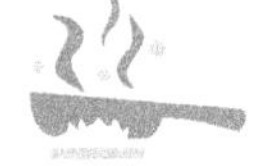

13 MINUTES

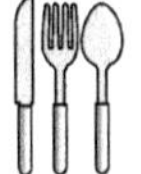

Servings:

2

Cranberries and fresh oranges in oatmeal? I can see you rolling your eyes. But it works!!! It is a fun way to bring excitement to an otherwise bland meal. The tart taste of the cranberries and the fresh, zesty freshness of the oranges not only improves the taste of the oatmeal but also adds extra vitamins and minerals to this healthy meal.

Nutritional Information per serving:

Total Carbs: 90.5g; Protein: 15.1g; Fat: 7.2g; Fibre: 12.9g; Sodium: 3mg; Calories:487

Ingredients:

- ½ cup of water
- 1 tbsp. of maple syrup
- 1 cup of freshly squeezed orange juice
- 1 tbsp. of freshly grated orange zest
- 1 cup of fresh cranberries
- 2 cups of gluten free rolled oats

Directions:

1. In a saucepan, mix the water, cranberries, and orange juice together and cook over medium heat. Allow it to cook for about 5 minutes.

2. Add the oats to the mix in the saucepan while occasionally stirring till it thickens. This should take about 8 minutes.

3. Take the saucepan off the burner and add the maple syrup while stirring gently.

4. Divide the oatmeal into two places and sprinkle in the orange zest.

5. Serve while hot.

Lemon and Raspberry Flavored Oatmeal Bars

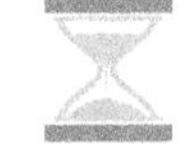

1H 30 MINUTES

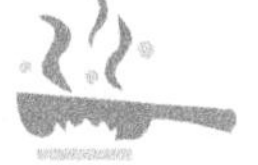

25 MINUTES

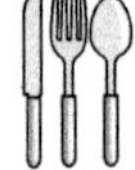

12 BARS

Not a lot of recipes are sweet and healthy. This oatmeal bar is one of the rare ones. Considerably healthy for a breakfast meal while also sweet enough to serve as dessert. This is a rare 2-in-1 combination. You can make them in advance and store them in the freezer. Whenever you need to, just whip them out, microwave, and have a sumptuous meal.

Nutritional Information per serving:

Total Carbs: 24.4g; Protein: 5.0g; Fat: 2.5g; Fibre: 4.4g; Sodium: 25mg; Calories:143

Ingredients:

- ¼ cup of pure maple syrup
- ½ tbsp. of vanilla extract (alcohol-free)
- ½ tbsp. of coconut sugar
- 1 large egg
- 1 ¼ cups of unsweetened almond milk
- 2 cups of fresh raspberries
- 2 tbsp. of freshly squeezed lemon juice
- 3 ½ cups of oats (fast cooking and gluten free)

Directions:

1. Heat the oven to about a temperature of 160 degrees Celsius.

2. Get a large clean bowl. Pour in the almond milk, egg, vanilla extract, maple syrup, and coconut sugar. Whisk thoroughly till they are well combined.

3. Add the raspberries, oats, and lemon juice to the mixture. Stir well till well combined.

4. Get a 9 x 13 inches baking dish and grease the inside with butter. Pour in the mixture and place in the oven for 25 minutes.

5. Once it is done, take it out of the oven and allow the baked oatmeal to cool for about one hour.

6. Cut the cooled oatmeal into 12 rectangular pieces, store in an airtight container and refrigerate.

7. To serve, thaw the oatmeal bars and serve warm. They can store for up to 3 days when refrigerated.

Scrambled Huevos Rancheros

Preparation time: 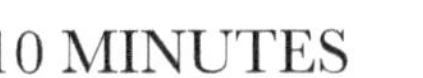 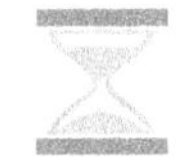	Cooking time: 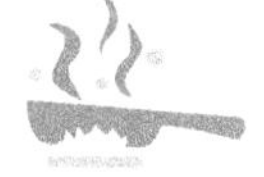 	Servings: 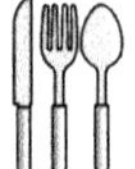
10 MINUTES	5 MINUTES	2

Are you craving a quick, super hearty breakfast meal? Are you short on time? Do you need extra protein? This scrambled egg—Mexican style is the answer you have been looking for. Do you need extra spice in it as well? Then serve with some sliced jalapenos.

Nutritional Information per serving:

Total Carbs: 6.9g; Protein: 13.3g; Fat: 15.6g; Fibre: 2.8g; Sodium: 956mg; Calories:239

Ingredients:

- ¼ tbsp. of freshly ground black pepper
- ¼ diced jalapenos (optional)
- ¼ cup of salsa (sugar-free)
- ¼ cup of diced fresh cilantro
- ½ tbsp. of salt
- 1 tbsp. of olive oil
- 4 large eggs

Ingredients for your homemade sugar free salsa

- 1/8 tbsp. of pepper
- ¼ tbsp. of salt
- ½ seeded jalapeno.
- 2 tomatoes
- 2 cilantro sprigs
- Freshly squeezed juice from half lemon

Directions:

1. In a medium sized bowl, whisk the pepper, eggs, and salt together.

2. Get a skillet over a burner on medium heat and add the olive oil. Allow the olive oil to heat up for 30 secs before pouring the egg mixture.

3. Scramble the egg mixture for about 4 minutes till it is well cooked.

4. Divide the scrambled eggs into two serving dishes and add the salsa, cilantro, and avocado.

5. Serve while hot.

To make the Salsa

1. Mix all the salsa ingredients in a bowl and transfer them into the food processor.

2. Allow it to run for about 4 minutes or until they are all thoroughly mixed.

3. Pour it out and store it in an airtight container for use at any time.

Cocoa flavored Smoothie with Toasted Coconut and Hazelnuts

10 MINUTES

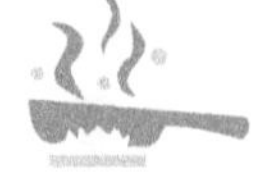

3 MINUTES

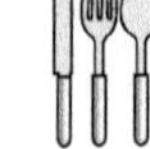

Servings:

1

A smoothie with healthy chocolate and nuts? That is one loaded breakfast chuck full of fats and nutrients. This is the perfect start to the day. Do you need it to be thicker? Just add more ice.

Nutritional Information per serving:

Total Carbs: 41.1g; Protein: 6.5g; Fat: 14.2g; Fibre: 6.6g; Sodium: 379mg; Calories:294

Ingredients:

- 1/8 tbsp. of seas salt
- 1 tbsp. of shelled pumpkin seeds
- 1 cup of unsweetened almond milk
- 1 tbsp. of diced unsweetened coconut
- 1 frozen ripe medium sized banana
- 1 ½ tbsp. of pure maple syrup
- 5 shelled and diced hazelnuts
- ½ cup of ice cubes

Directions:

1. Get a skillet over a burner on medium heat. Pour in the diced coconut and keep stirring till you get a golden-brown coloration of them. After the diced coconut is toasted for about 3 minutes, pour it into a plate and set aside.

2. In a blender, add the cocoa powder, salt, maple syrup, banana, milk, and ice, then blend together until you get a smooth consistency. If you want the smoothie to be thicker, add more ice and blend. You should get a smooth consistency in about 3 minutes.

3. Pour the blended smoothie into a serving bowl. Add the toasted coconut, hazelnuts, and pumpkin seeds and serve.

Oats spiced with Almond Butter pumpkin

Preparation time: 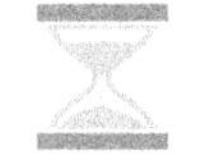
8 H (OVERNIGHT)

Cooking time: 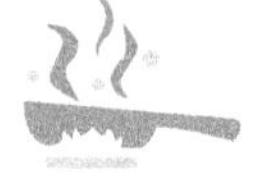 
0 MINUTES

Servings: 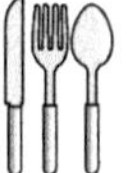
2

This is an amazing meal to have during a busy day. The deliciousness of these Oats would leave you feeling full and satisfied all through the day.

Nutritional Information per serving:

Total Carbs: 30.4g; Protein: 8.4g; Fat: 14.9g; Fibre: 5.9g; Sodium: 25mg; Calories:288

Ingredients:

- ¼ cup of pumpkin puree
- ¼ cup of unsweetened almond milk
- ½ cup of gluten free rolled oats
- ½ tbsp. of ground cinnamon
- ½ tbsp. of pumpkin pie spice
- ½ tbsp. of alcohol-free vanilla extract
- 1 tbsp. of pure maple syrup
- 2 tbsp. of diced walnuts
- 2 tbsp. of sugar free, unsalted almond butter

Directions:

1. Get a large bowl to mix the milk and oats. Add the cinnamon, vanilla extract, maple syrup, pumpkin pie spice, and pumpkin puree. Mix everything thoroughly.

2. Get two small canning jars. Pour half of the mixture into each jar and add one tablespoonful of the unsalted almond butter on top.

3. Cover each of the jars with their lid and refrigerate overnight.

4. Add the walnut to the refrigerated mixture in the morning and serve. The mix would last for 3 days if properly refrigerated.

Baked Apples with Skin

20 MINUTES 

15 MINUTES 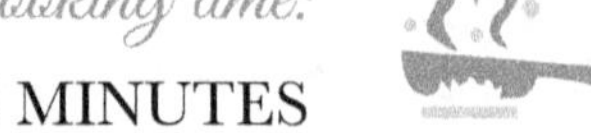

3 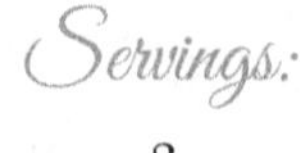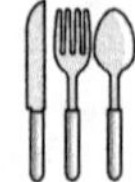

A sweet-tasting natural meal with no additional sweeteners, the skin on the apples provides extra fiber for your guts—an overall pleasing breakfast dish.

Nutritional Information per serving:

Total Carbs: 31.3g; Protein: 1.4g; Fat: 8.0g; Fibre: 7.5g; Sodium: 2mg; Calories:203

Ingredients:

- 1 cup of diced unsweetened coconut
- 1 tbsp. of ground cinnamon
- 6 pieces of Pink Lady Apples.

Directions:

1. Remove the core from the apples to about half an inch from the bottom of the apple. Take care to keep the apple hollow as such.

2. Fill the hollowed center of the apple with the diced coconut with the cinnamon sprinkled on it. Once you have filled all the apples, place them on a baking sheet.

3. Preheat the oven to about 160 degrees Celsius and bake the apples for about 15 minutes.

4. Once the Apples are soft and brown at the top, take them from the oven and serve hot.

Kale spiced Scrambled Eggs

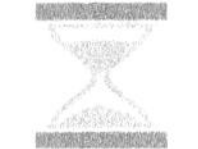

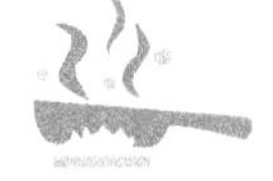

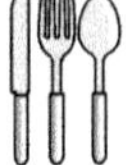

With extra proteins and green veggies, the Scramble is a great breakfast choice. It is a great meal choice after an awesome morning workout.

Nutritional Information per serving:

Total Carbs: 7.0g; Protein: 20.2g; Fat: 26.5g; Fibre: 2.1g; Sodium: 1,382mg; Calories:359

Ingredients:

- 1/8 tbsp. of ground cayenne pepper
- ¼ tbsp. of freshly ground black pepper
- ½ tbsp. of salt
- 1 cup of fresh diced kale
- 1 tbsp. of olive oil
- 2 tbsp. of ground turmeric
- 3 large eggs

Directions:

1. Break the eggs into a bowl. Add the turmeric, black pepper, cayenne pepper, and salt to the eggs. Whisk thoroughly till they are well combined. Set aside.

2. Get a skillet over a burner on medium heat. Add the olive oil and heat for about one minute.

3. Add the Kale to the heated olive oil and cook for about 3 minutes till it is wilted.

4. Add the mixed egg to the Kale and scramble the eggs until it is well cooked.

5. You can also add spinach, collard greens to the kale for extra nutritious veggies.

6. Serve hot.

Chicken Sausage Patty

 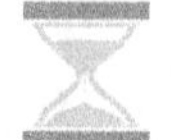
15 MINUTES

Cooking time: 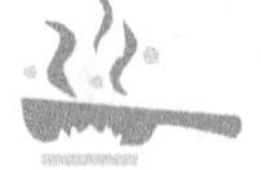
10 MINUTES

Servings: 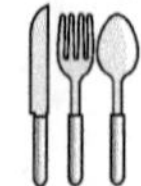
24 PATTIES

Our patties are well balanced. With a healthy dose of protein, fat, and low carb, this is one healthy meal you can't afford to miss. You can serve this with a well-made vegetarian hash (recipe below) or poached eggs.

Nutritional Information per serving:

Total Carbs: 1.0g; Protein: 10.1g; Fat: 6.4g; Fibre: 0.2g; Sodium: 35mg; Calories:105

Ingredients:

- ½ cup of finely diced fresh flat-leaf parsley
- 1 tbsp. of fresh minced ginger
- 1 tbsp. of ground white pepper
- 1 tbsp. of diced fresh sage
- 1 tbsp. of ground cloves
- 1 medium sized diced yellow onion
- 2 tbsp. of red pepper flakes
- 3 pounds of ground chicken
- 4 tbsp. of olive oil
- 6 diced garlic cloves

Directions:

1. Get a large bowl. Mix the clove, diced onions, ginger, garlic, and chicken together. Then add the remaining ingredients and mix thoroughly, leaving out the olive oil.

2. Mold the mixture into 24 2-inch sized round patties.

3. Get a large sauté pan over the burner on medium heat and heat the olive oil for 30 seconds.

4. Place the patties into the oil and sauté till it is well cooked. This would take you about 10 minutes to sauté both sides.

Quinoa Pizza Muffins

Preparation time:		Cooking time:		Servings:
45 MINUTES	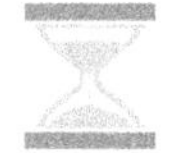	40 MINUTES	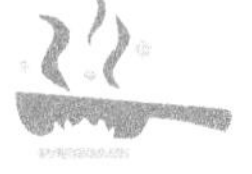	12 MUFFINS 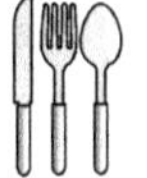

We know the all too popular English muffin pizzas. This is a healthier sugar free spin on your favorite English muffin. Do you have 35-40 minutes to spare? This is the meal for you.

Nutritional Information per serving:

Total Carbs: 12.1g; Protein: 6.7g; Fat: 4.4g; Fibre: 1.6g; Sodium: 278mg; Calories:119

Ingredients:

- ¼ cup of fresh diced basil
- ½ cup of fresh cut spinach
- ½ tbsp. of salt
- ½ tbsp. of freshly ground black pepper
- 1 cup of rinsed uncooked quinoa
- 1 tbsp. of dried oregano
- 1 ½ cups of sugar free marinara sauce
- 2 cups of water
- 2 large eggs

Directions:

1. Boil the quinoa with water in a saucepan on high heat. Then reduce the heat to low and allow the quinoa to simmer for about 15 minutes. Once it is tender, off the heat and set aside.

2. Break the eggs in a bowl and whisk thoroughly. Add the whisked eggs and the cheese, spinach, salt, oregano, pepper, and basil to the tender quinoa. Mix them till they are well combined.

3. Lubricate the inside of a 12-cup muffin tin with the cooking spray. Then pour the mixture into the muffin tin, careful not to fill it to the brim. Gently press it down with your fingers or a spoon.

4. Preheat the oven to 160 degrees Celsius and bake the muffins for approximately 20 minutes.

5. Once it is done, take it out and allow it to cool for another 5 minutes.

6. Serve with warm marinara sauce on top.

Cheese and Artichoke Squares

Preparation time: 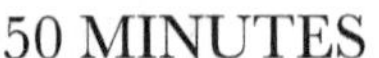 	Cooking time: 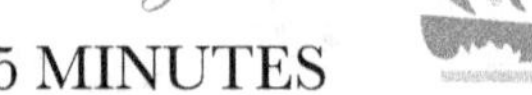 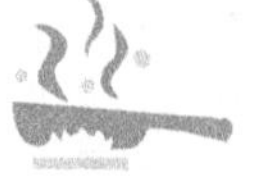	Servings: 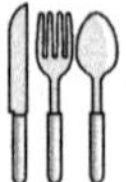
50 MINUTES	35 MINUTES	2

These healthy squares are high in protein and sodium. They are quite easy to prepare and can be made well ahead of time.

Nutritional Information per serving:

Total Carbs: 5.5g; Protein: 12.1g; Fat: 11.2g; Fibre: 2.3g; Sodium: 665mg; Calories:175

Ingredients:

- ¼ tbsp. of tabasco
- ¼ tbsp. of freshly ground black pepper
- ¼ tbsp. of ground dried oregano
- ½ tbsp. of salt
- 1 shredded small sized yellow onion
- 1 jar of chopped drained and marinated artichoke hearts with the liquid
- 2 tbsp. of fresh chopped flat-leaf parsley
- 2 tbsp. of coconut flour
- 2 shredded garlic cloves
- 4 large eggs
- 8 ounces of finely chopped Monterey jack cheese

Directions:

1. Preheat the oven to a temperature of about 160 degrees Celsius.

2. Break the eggs in a medium sized bowl and whisk very well. Add the flour, tabasco, oregano, pepper, and salt and mix well. Set the mixture aside.

3. Get a skillet over the burner on medium heat and heat up the artichoke liquid for about 1 minute. Set it aside.

4. In a skillet as well, and over medium heat, saute the onions and garlic for another 5 minutes.

5. Add the cheese, parsley, onion, garlic, and artichoke to the egg mix. Combine them thoroughly.

6. Pour the mixture into an ungreased baking dish and bake for about 30 minutes. Once the egg is set, take it out of the oven and allow it to cool for 10 minutes.

7. Cut it into squares and serve warm.

Small Baked Eggplant Pizza bites

Preparation time: 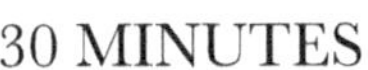
30 MINUTES 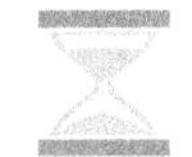

Cooking time: 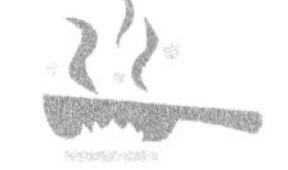
25 MINUTES

Servings: 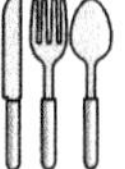
1

An easy to make Eggplant Pizza bite. Gluten free with a good, healthy fat. This would preferably serve as a quick snack on the go.

Nutritional Information per serving:

Total Carbs: 19.5g; Protein: 9.0g; Fat: 16.5g; Fibre: 9.3g; Sodium: 322mg; Calories:247

Ingredients:

- ½ tbsp. of salt
- ½ cup of marinara sauce
- ¼ cup of shredded mozzarella cheese
- 2 tbsp. of dried oregano
- 2 large eggs
- 2 tbsp. of olive oil
- 2 medium sized eggplants
- ¾ cup of almond meal

Directions:

1. Preheat the oven to a temperature of about 205 degrees Celsius.

2. Cut the eggplants into square shapes by cutting off the circles on the sides. Place them in a colander and sprinkle with salt. Toss them in the colander and allow them to sit for 10 minutes before rinsing with water.

3. Get a small bowl. Add the oregano and the almond meal in it and stir till they are well mixed.

4. In another bowl, break the eggs in and whisk them thoroughly.

5. Take the square-shaped eggplant and dip it in the egg. Take it out and tap off excess eggs, then dip in the oregano mixture. Place the dipped eggplant on a non-stick baking sheet.

6. Pour the olive oil lightly over the dipped eggplants and bake in the oven for 12 minutes.

7. Take out the baking sheet. Scoop some marinara sauce on the eggplants and sprinkle the shredded mozzarella on top. Bake for another 2 minutes or until the cheese has melted.

8. Serve while hot.

Zucchini Noodles with Pesto

Preparation time: 10 MINUTES  | **Cooking time:** 5 MINUTES 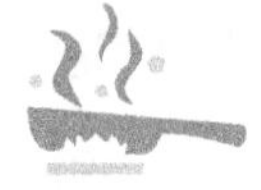 | **Servings:** 1 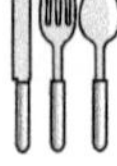

Zoodles, as they are fondly called, are a healthy pasta meal. It is fun and easy to make.

Nutritional Information per serving:

Total Carbs: 9.6g; Protein: 40.4g; Fat: 42.5g; Fibre: 2.5g; Sodium: 875mg; Calories:606

Ingredients:

- ¾ cup of fresh basil leaves
- ¼ cup of pine nuts
- 1 pound of Zucchini
- ½ cup of freshly grated parmesan cheese
- 2 tbsp. of garlic-infused olive oil
- ¼ tbsp. of sea salt
- 3 tbsp. of olive oil
- ¼ tbsp. of freshly ground black pepper

Directions:

1. Get a large bowl. Peel the zucchini into long narrow ribbons. Set aside.

2. Heat one tablespoon of olive oil in a sauté pan over medium heat for about a minute. Add the zucchini noodles, half portion of the black pepper, and half portion of the salt. Continue to stir it in the sauté pan for approx. Five minutes till the Zucchini noodles are tender.

3. To prepare the pesto sauce. Add the basil, garlic infused oil, basil, and pine nuts into the food processor and pulse them till they are coarsely mixed. Add the remaining ingredients to the food processor and run it till all the ingredients are smooth and well combined.

4. Serve the hot cooked zucchini noodles with the pesto sauce.

Cranberry Almond Granola

Preparation time: 25 MINUTES 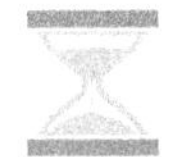

Cooking time: 20 MINUTES 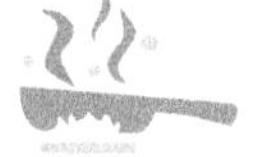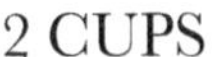

Servings: 2 CUPS 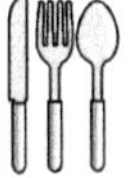

A snack, you may call it. Others would take it as a meal with almond or coconut milk or even yogurt. The cranberry almond granola is that versatile.

Nutritional Information per serving:

Total Carbs: 11.4g; Protein: 1.9g; Fat: 5.8g; Fibre: 1.6g; Sodium: 1mg; Calories:105

Ingredients:

- ¼ tbsp. of vanilla extract, alcohol free
- ¼ tbsp. of almond extract, alcohol free
- ½ tbsp. of ground cinnamon
- 1 tbsp. of flaxseeds
- 1 cup of rolled oats, gluten free
- 1 tbsp. of whole walnuts
- 1 tbsp. of slivered almonds
- 2 tbsp. of dried cranberries, sugar free
- 3 tbsp. of pure maple syrup
- 3 tbsp. of melted coconut oil

Directions:

1. Get a bowl to mix the oil, almond extract, maple syrup, and vanilla extract. Then set it aside.

2. Preheat the oven to 160 degrees Celsius.

3. Ground the walnuts in a blender and transfer them into a large bowl. Pour the flaxseed into the bender and ground till it is smooth and add to the walnut in the bowl.

4. Add the cinnamon, almonds, and oats to the walnut bowl and mix thoroughly.

5. Pour the oil and maple syrup mix on the walnut mixture and stir to combine.

6. On an ungreased baking sheet, spread out the granola and bake in the oven for 15 minutes. Stir constantly till the granola is light brown.

7. Remove the granola from the oven and add the cranberries to it. Stir well to ensure an even mix. Then serve warm.

8. You can also transfer the granola and cranberries into an airtight container. This can be refrigerated for up to 3 weeks. You can bring it out and warm it in 5 minutes for a ready meal.

Bacon and Vegetable Omelet

<table>
<tr>
<td>
20 MINUTES</td>
<td>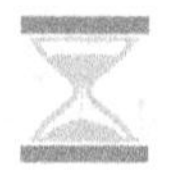</td>
<td>
15 MINUTES</td>
<td>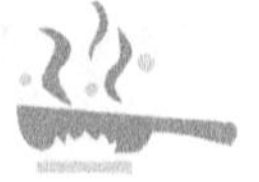</td>
<td>
2</td>
<td>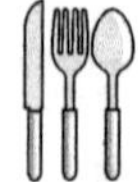</td>
</tr>
</table>

Everybody eats bacon and eggs. It has become a staple in our diet. It is quick and easy to prepare. Adding a vegetable to this breakfast tradition is a sure way to ensure that you have all the nutrients you need to get started for the day.

Nutritional Information per serving:

Total Carbs: 9.6g; Protein: 40.4g; Fat: 42.5g; Fibre: 2.5g; Sodium: 875mg; Calories:606

Ingredients:

- ¼ cup of chopped fresh basil leaves
- 1 cup of white mushrooms, sliced
- 1 medium size chopped zucchini
- 1 medium sized chopped yellow summer squash
- 2 tbsp. of olive oil
- 6 slices of diced nitrate free bacon
- 8 large eggs

Directions:

1. Cook the bacon in a large sauté pan on medium high heat for 5 minutes until it is crispy. Add the basil and vegetables to the bacon and sauté for about 8 minutes till they are tender.

2. Break the eggs into a bowl and mix thoroughly. Set the whisked eggs aside.

3. Get another sauté pan over medium heat and heat the olive oil for about one minute. Add the eggs to the oil and cook on each side for about 3 minutes.

4. Pour the sauteed veggies and bacon on one half of the egg. Then fold the second half of the egg over the veggies to form a vegetable filling.

5. Serve hot.

Stuffed Eggs

<table>
<tr><td>Preparation time:
20 MINUTES</td><td>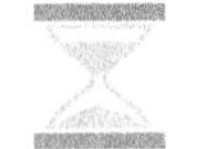</td><td>Cooking time:
15 MINUTES</td><td>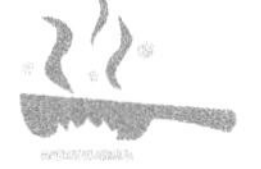</td><td>Servings:
4</td><td>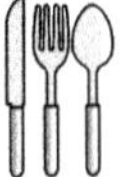</td></tr>
</table>

Stuffed Eggs are an amazing appetizer before the main meal. It can also serve as an aside to a salad meal. The confluence of flavors in this dish would amaze you.

Nutritional Information per serving:

Total Carbs: 1.9g; Protein: 7.1g; Fat: 12.3g; Fibre: 0.1g; Sodium: 340mg; Calories:161

Ingredients:

- ¼ tbsp. of salt
- ¼ tbsp. of grass fed unsalted butter
- ¼ tbsp. of ground white pepper
- ¼ cup of Dijon mustard
- 1 tbsp. of fresh chives, chopped
- 1 tbsp. of fresh tarragon, chopped
- 1 tbsp. of rice wine vinegar
- 2 tbsp. of well-diced shallots
- 3 tbsp. of full fat coconut milk, unsweetened
- 8 large eggs

Directions:

1. Set your oven broiler to low and get it going.
2. Boil the eggs in a pot till they are hard boiled. Take out the eggs and peel the shells off. Slice each egg in half lengthwise and set aside.
3. Take out the yolks from the eggs and transfer them into a bowl. Mix with the milk, shallots, vinegar, chives, mustard, and tarragon with the egg yolks till they are well combined. Add the pepper and salt to season.
4. With a spoon, scoop the egg mixture into the hollow sections of the egg whites. If you have a piping bag, piping the mixture into the egg whites would also do the trick.
5. Brush the top of the eggs with butter and place them in a baking dish. Broil the eggs in the oven for approximately 5 minutes till they are lightly browned at the top.
6. Remove the eggs from the oven and serve warm.

Salmon Omelet

 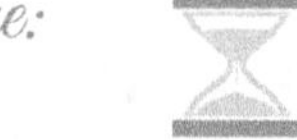
30 MINUTES

Cooking time: 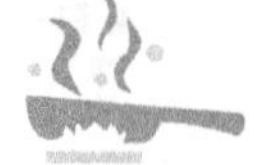
24 MINUTES

Servings: 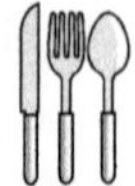
2

A breakfast meal with an abundance of mega-3 fatty acids, the salmon omelet breakfast with its high protein, high fat, and low carb content would have you feeling satisfied and full of energy throughout the day.

Nutritional Information per serving:

Total Carbs: 4.6g; Protein: 42.9g; Fat: 30.2g; Fibre: 1.7g; Sodium: 544mg; Calories:484

Ingredients:

- ¼ cup of trimmed scallions, chopped
- 1 cup of trimmed asparagus, chopped
- 1 tbsp. of fresh chopped dill
- 2 tbsp. of olive oil
- 6 ounces of canned salmon
- 6 large eggs

Directions:

1. Place a skillet over a burner on medium high heat and add the dill, olive oil, asparagus, and scallions. Sauté the mixture for close to 10 minutes till the asparagus is visibly soft. Remove the skillet from the burner. Transfer the mixture to a plate and set aside.

2. Return the skillet back on the burner, still on medium high heat. Depending on how thick the salmon is, sauté the salmon for about 10-15 minutes. Once the salmon is flaky, remove the skillet from the burner and transfer the content to another plate.

3. Break the eggs into a bowl and whisk thoroughly. Clean the skillet with a paper towel and place it back on the burner. Pour the whisked eggs into the skillet and allow the eggs to cook. Ideally, you cook the eggs for 4 minutes on both sides till they are light brown.

4. Once the eggs are done, transfer them to a plate. On one half of the egg, place the asparagus mix and the salmon the fold over the other half of the egg to form a closed filling.

5. Serve warm.

Onion Jam

55 MINUTES 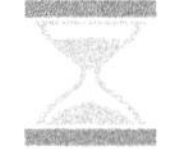

45 MINUTES 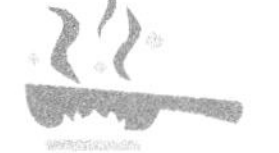

1 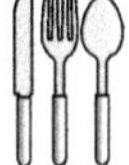

Sweet tasting carefully prepared caramelized onion jam, a perfect addition to your cookies and crackers. The complex natural flavor from this jam is a savory delight to your palate.

Nutritional Information per serving:

Total Carbs: 14.0g; Protein: 1.7g; Fat: 3.4g; Fibre: 2.6g; Sodium: 151mg; Calories:89

Ingredients:

- ½ tbsp. of salt
- 2 sprigs of fresh thyme without the stems
- 2 tbsp. of olive oil
- 8 large white onions

Directions:

1. Carefully peel and slice the onions thinly across the grain.

2. Get the burner on medium heat. Heat the olive oil for a minute in a heavy bottomed pan. Once the oil starts to shimmer, add the onions and thyme and stir. Add salt to season.

3. Lower the heat and continue to stir the onions till it starts caramelizing. While you continue to stir, keep scraping the dried onion juices with a spoon, mixing it with the onions. Do this repeatedly for about 40 minutes till you get sufficient thick spread onion juices. This slow heating method breaks down the onions gradually, ensuring that you get all the flavors present in them.

4. Turn off the burner and allow it to cool down to room temperature.

5. Serve warm with your sugar free crackers.

Preparation time: 
35 MINUTES

Cooking time: 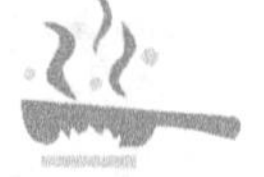
30 MINUTES

Servings: 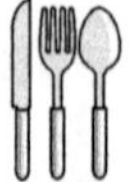
1

The vegetarian hash is a wonderful dessert and can also be taken as a side to the main dish. It is a healthy spin on the familiar hash coupled with its awesome pleasant taste.

Nutritional Information per serving:

Total Carbs: 26.2g; Protein: 2.9g; Fat: 0.9g; Fibre: 3.7g; Sodium: 143mg; Calories:119

Ingredients:

- ¼ tbsp. of salt
- ¼ tbsp. of freshly cracked peppercorns, black
- ¼ bunch of chopped cilantro leaves
- ½ tbsp. of olive oil
- I tbsp. of chili pepper
- 1 sliced medium sized red onion
- 1 ½ pound of diced russet potatoes
- 2 sliced and seeded medium sized red bell peppers

Directions:

1. Preheat the oven to a temperature of 205 degrees Celsius

2. Pour the onions, pepper, and potatoes into a medium sized bowl. Toss them in olive oil, then drain the oil from them on a rack.

3. Pour the tossed vegetables into an ungreased baking sheet. Season with peppercorns and chili powder. Roast the seasoned vegetables in the oven for 30 minutes till it is tender before taking it out of the oven

4. Add the cilantro and season with salt. Serve warm.

Tomatoes with Mushroom Stuffing

Preparation time: 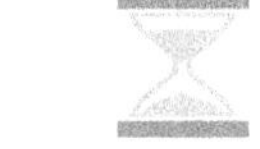
1 HOUR

Cooking time: 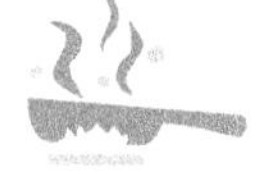
50 MINUTES

Servings: 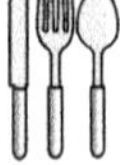
2

Beautiful flavors of the mushrooms mixed with the sweet plump juices from Roma tomatoes would give you a great culinary delight. Perfect breakfast for a perfect day.

Nutritional Information per serving:

Total Carbs: 9.3g; Protein: 4.2g; Fat: 6.4g; Fibre: 2.7g; Sodium: 495mg; Calories:106

Ingredients:

- ¼ cup of white wine
- ¼ tbsp. freshly ground black pepper
- ¼ cup of finely diced flat-leaf parsley
- 1 pound of white mushroom
- 1 ¼ tbsp. of salt
- 2 tbsp. of olive oil
- 3 tbsp. of almond meal
- 4 finely chopped medium sized shallots
- 6 large ripe Roma tomatoes.

Directions:

1. Preheat the oven to a temperature of 180 degrees Celsius.
2. Cut the mushroom into small pieces. Place them into the food processor in batches to pulse for about 5 minutes each to prevent the mushrooms from clumping. Pulse all the mushrooms till they are finely chopped. Set aside.
3. Cut the Roma tomatoes crosswise. Then trim the rounded end flat. Remove the innards from the tomatoes. Rub the insides of the hollowed-out tomatoes with salt and set them aside.
4. Place a large skillet over medium heat. Sauté the shallots with 1 tablespoon of olive oil for one minute. Include the finely chopped mushrooms. Season with salt and increase the heat to high.
5. Continue to cook till there are no more moisture in the mushrooms, then add white wine and cook for 5 more minutes. When most of the wine has evaporated, turn off the burner. Add in the parsley, the pepper, and stir.
6. Scoop the mushroom filling into the tomatoes till it bulges slightly and sprinkle the top with the almond meal.
7. Arrange the stuffed tomatoes in an ungreased baking dish and drizzle the tops with the left-over olive oil. Bake the tomato fillings for 25 minutes till they become soft.
8. Remove from the oven and serve hot.

Roasted Beets

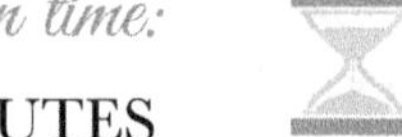

Preparation time:

1 H 15 MINUTES

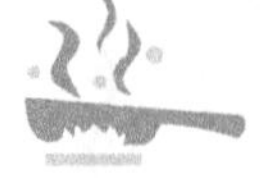

Cooking time:

1 HOUR

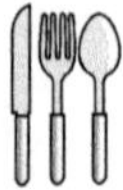

Servings:

2

Sweet, if you find yourself craving sugary foods or you have a tendency to binge on unhealthy food, the roasted beets are for you. It has an amazing capacity to stop your body from craving sugar. Roasting has been a sure-fire way of bringing out the sweet natural juices in the beets and caramelizing them on the surface to give that satisfying crunch.

Nutritional Information per serving:

Total Carbs: 8.3g; Protein: 1.4g; Fat: 1.7g; Fibre: 2.5g; Sodium: 139mg; Calories:52

Ingredients:

- ¼ tbsp. of salt
- ¼ tbsp. of fresh chopped flat-leaf parsley
- ¼ tbsp. of ground cinnamon
- 1 tbsp. of Olive oil
- 2 pounds of beets

Directions:

1. Cut the beets into 1-inch wedges in a bowl. Sprinkle the beets with the olive oil, add the cinnamon and the salt. Toss them in the bowl and set them aside.

2. Preheat the oven to a temperature of 180 degrees Celsius.

3. In the middle rack of the oven, roast the beets till they are soft. This would take about an hour. Ensure you turn them every 30 minutes when you are roasting.

4. Remove from the oven and sprinkle the roasted beets with the chopped parsley. Serve hot.

Lamb Patties

Preparation time: 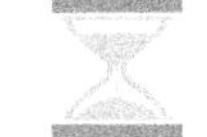
20 MINUTES

Cooking time: 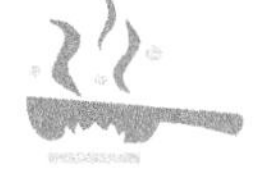
15 MINUTES

Servings: 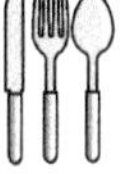
3

The trick to this dish is to ensure that the eggs are well cooked while the lamb is medium-rare or rare done. You can serve them with chia seed jam (recipe above) or even a fruit chutney (the cranberry chutney recipe above).

Nutritional Information per serving:

Total Carbs: 21.4g; Protein: 27.3g; Fat: 21.8g; Fibre: 3.6g; Sodium: 243mg; Calories:399

Ingredients:

- 1/8 tbsp. of salt
- ¼ tbsp. of black peppercorns, freshly cracked
- ¼ cup of dried currants
- ¼ cup of whole pistachio nuts
- ½ tbsp. of ground cinnamon
- ½ pound of ground lamb
- 1 medium minced shallot
- 2 cloves of minced garlic

Directions:

1. Preheat the oven to a temperature of 180 degrees Celsius.
2. Mix all the ingredients in a bowl till they are well combined.
3. Mold the mixture into six pieces of small ovals.
4. Place the molds in a baking dish and bake in the oven for 15 minutes. Serve warm.

Eggplant Parmigiana

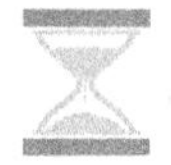

40 MINUTES

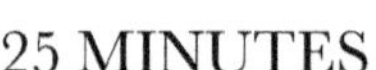
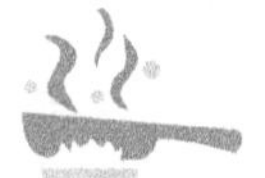

25 MINUTES

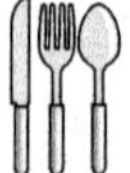

1

This is a much healthier version of your grandma's recipe. It is a gluten free twist with the flour and almond meal giving you a nice full feel on every bite.

Nutritional Information per serving:

Total Carbs: 34.7g; Protein: 42.5g; Fat: 41.9g; Fibre: 16.3g; Sodium: 1,672mg; Calories: 680

Ingredients:

- ¼ cup of olive oil, divided into two parts
- ½ cup of water
- 1 cup of coconut four
- 1 tbsp. of fresh chopped flat leaf parsley
- 1 medium thinly sliced eggplant
- 1 pound of shredded mozzarella cheese
- 1 jar of tomato sauce, sugar free
- 3 cups of almond meal
- 3 large eggs

Directions:

1. Preheat the oven to a temperature of 180 degrees Celsius.

2. Break the eggs into a bowl and mix thoroughly with water. Set aside.

3. Get two more bowls. In one, pour in the almond meal and pour the flour in another bowl.

4. Take one slice of the eggplant and dip it inside the flour; shake it to get rid of the excess flour. Dip that same slice in the egg mixture and shake to get rid of the excess. Do the same for the almond meal shaking the slice to rid the excess almond meal on it. Once you are done dipping the slice in the 3 bowls, set it aside. Do the same for all the eggplant slices.

5. Get a medium size skillet on a burner on medium heat. Heat 2 tablespoons of olive oil in the skillet for one minute. Increase the heat to medium high and fry the eggplant slices in it till both sides turn golden. Drain the fried eggplants on a paper towel.

6. Arrange the fried eggplants on an ungreased baking dish. Add a tablespoon of tomato sauce and one small heap of shredded mozzarella cheese. Bake the slices for 15 minutes till the cheese melts.

7. Take the baked eggplants from the oven and garnish with parsley and to the leftover tomato sauce.

Pork and Fennel Meatballs

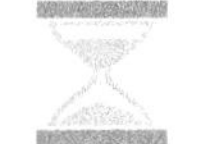

Preparation time:
35 MINUTES

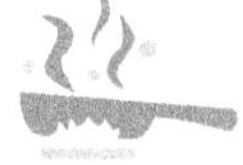

Cooking time:
25 MINUTES

Servings:
24 MEATBALLS

You can eat the meatballs with marinara sauce or pasta. Or you could just choose to have them like that as an entrée. Meatballs are always a yummy, delicious option in your meal.

Nutritional Information per serving:

Total Carbs: 0.3g; Protein: 3.9g; Fat: 4.1g; Fibre: 0.2g; Sodium: 38mg; Calories:54

Ingredients:

- ¼ tbsp. of salt
- ½ tbsp. of freshly ground black pepper
- 1 pound of 84% lean ground pork
- 1 large egg
- 1 ½ tbsp. of olive oil
- 2 tbsp. of fennel seeds
- 2 tbsp. of fresh flat leaf parsley, roughly chopped
- 3 tbsp. of almond meal

Directions:

1. Mix the parsley, pork, salt, egg, pepper, and almond meal in a bowl till they are well combined. Mold the mixture into 24 1-inch sized meatballs.

2. Heat the olive oil in a skillet over medium heat for 1 minute. Sauté the fennel seeds in the fillet till the aroma comes out. That should take about 4 minutes tops.

3. Add the meatballs to the skillet and brown them on all the sides for 20 minutes. You would know the meatballs are cooked through when there is no pink on the inside. Serve hot.

Marinated London Broil

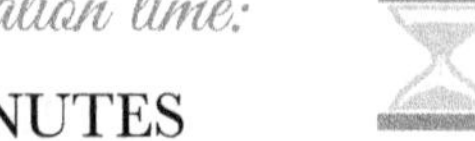

Preparation time: 20 MINUTES

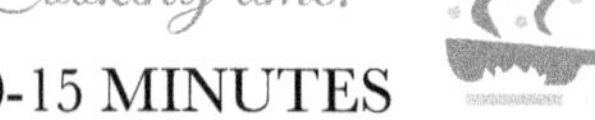

Cooking time: 10-15 MINUTES

Servings: 1

We all know there is nothing quite like the natural juices from grilled meat. With a rub made from cloves and cinnamon, you would have a delicious tasting steak quite like nothing you have tasted.

Nutritional Information per serving:

Total Carbs: 1.0g; Protein: 24.6g; Fat: 5.7g; Fibre: 0.4g; Sodium: 159mg; Calories:170

Ingredients:

- ¼ tbsp. of salt
- ¼ tbsp. of black peppercorns, freshly cracked
- ½ tbsp. of ground cloves
- 1 tbsp. of ground cumin
- 1 cup of dry red wine
- 1 tbsp. of olive oil
- 1 tbsp. of ground cinnamon
- 1 ½ pound of London broil

Directions:

1. Preheat the grill with the setting on medium heat.
2. Boil the London broil in a pot till it is done. Take it out and cut it across the grain. Then, set it aside
3. Mix the oil, seasoning, and wine in a small bowl.
4. Cover the meat with the mixture and grill it in the oven till it is done to your taste.
5. Slice the meat and serve.

Mushroom Pork Medallions

 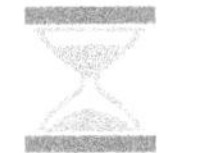
40 MINUTES

Cooking time: 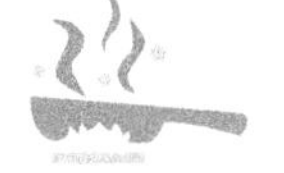
25-30 MINUTES

Servings: 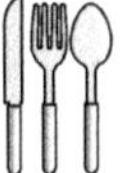
2

Our delicious, gluten free pork medallions with the mushrooms are so packed with antioxidants and omega-3 fatty acids. The flax meal especially adds that nutty flavor we all love.

Nutritional Information per serving:

Total Carbs: 5.8g; Protein: 40.7g; Fat: 13.2g; Fibre: 1.3g; Sodium: 433mg; Calories:311

Ingredients:

- 1/8 tbsp. of freshly ground black pepper
- ¼ tbsp. of crushed dried rosemary
- ¼ cup of white mushroom, sliced
- ½ cup of beef broth, no salt added
- 1 sliced small sized yellow onion
- 1 tbsp. of olive oil
- 1 pound of sliced tenderloin, ½ inch size thick medallion
- 1 clove of minced garlic
- 2 tbsp. of flax meal

Directions:

1. Heat the olive oil in a large skillet over medium heat for 30 seconds. Brown the pork in the skillet till it is brown on each side. Once it is done, remove the pork from the skillet and set it aside.

2. Using the same skillet as before, sauté the garlic, onions, and mushroom for about a minute. Add the flax meal and stir it until It is well blended.

3. Pour in the broth and stir gently. Add in the pepper and the rosemary. Increase the heat to high and cook till it boils. Continue to stir the broth till it becomes thick.

4. Put the pork medallion on the mixture that is in the skillet. Get the burner back to low and allow the meat to simmer for 15 minutes. This would allow the juices in the medallion to run. Then serve hot.

Peppers stuffed with Lentils

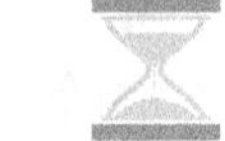

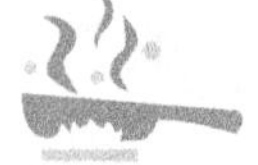

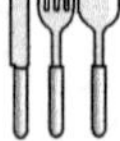

You can make these stuffed peppers and just save them in your refrigerator. You can then just bring them out for a quick breakfast anytime you want to eat them.

Nutritional Information per serving:

Total Carbs: 75.3g; Protein: 28.3g; Fat: 7.8g; Fibre: 14.3g; Sodium: 745mg; Calories:473

Ingredients:

- ¼ tbsp. of black pepper, freshly cracked
- 1 tbsp. of olive oil
- 2 medium sized diced yellow onions
- 2 finely diced large carrots
- 2 finely diced medium celery stalks
- 3 cups of dried red lentils
- 3 ounces of feta cheese
- 4 cups of vegetable stock
- 6 sprigs of fresh oregano
- 6 medium sized red bell peppers

Directions:

1. Get a saucepot and place it on medium heat, pour in the olive oil, and heat for 1 minute. Sauté the carrots, onions, and celery for 5 minutes. Add one cup of the vegetable stock and the lentils. Let it simmer for 20 minutes till the lentils are cooked.

2. Chop the oregano leaves and reserve the tops. Set it aside.

3. Seed the bell pepper, cut off the tops, and remove the ribs as well. Place them in a pot with three cups of the vegetable stock and allow to simmer for 10 minutes on medium heat with the pot covered.

4. Get a large bowl and mix the feta, black peppercorns, chopped oregano, and the lentil mix we prepared earlier. Then fill the bell peppers with the mixture.

5. With the stem tops open, serve the peppers and garnish them with the remaining oregano tops.

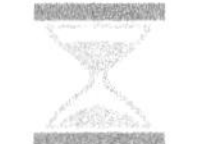
4 H 30 MINUTES

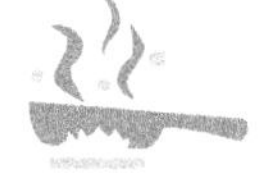
16 MINUTES

2

Citrus flavored steak is a rare delicacy. It is better served with garden salad and garnished with blueberries or even strawberries for that fruity kick.

Nutritional Information per serving:

Total Carbs: 0.3g; Protein: 16.3g; Fat: 27.5g; Fibre: 0.0g; Sodium: 52mg; Calories:333

Ingredients:

- ¼ tbsp. of salt
- ¼ cup of toasted sesame oil
- ¼ tbsp. of freshly ground black pepper
- 1 tbsp. of pure maple syrup
- 1 tbsp. of pineapple juice
- 1 tbsp. of freshly squeezed lime juice
- 1 flank steak
- 1 5-inch sized thinly sliced ginger knob
- 2 tbsp. of olive oil

Directions:

1. Put the maple syrup, salt, sesame oil, lime juice, ginger, pineapple juice, and pepper in the food processor and run it till you get a smooth consistency. After about thirty seconds, get the content out of the processor and into a bowl.

2. Put the steak in the same bowl. Make sure it is totally covered with the mixture. Cover to marinade and refrigerate it for 4 hours.

3. With a cast iron skillet, heat the olive oil over medium heat for about a minute.

4. Cook the steak in the skillet for 8 minutes on each side. Place the steak, covered with foil on a cutting board and allow it to rest for 10 minutes.

5. Slice the steak perpendicular to the grain and serve warm.

Fish Curry

Preparation time: 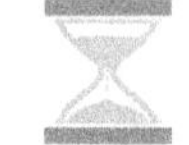
45 MINUTES

Cooking time: 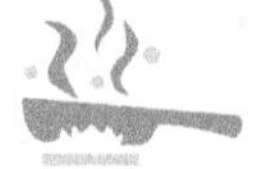
40 MINUTES

Servings: 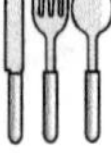
1

The spices we have incorporated into this curry and the wild salmon provide our body with the essential fat and proteins we need to keep a healthy body. Of special importance is the omega-3 that is abundant in the fish added to this curry.

Nutritional Information per serving:

Total Carbs: 15.2g; Protein: 29.7g; Fat: 45.5g; Fibre: 3.8g; Sodium: 1,086mg; Calories:592

Ingredients:

- ½ tbsp. of ground turmeric
- ¼ tbsp. of ground cumin
- ¼ tbsp. of fish sauce, gluten free
- ¼ tbsp. of grated ginger
- ¼ tbsp. of ground coriander
- ½ diced small stalk celery
- ½ pound of wild salmon with the skin removed
- 1 tbsp. of curry powder
- 1 chopped medium sized carrot
- 2 tbsp. of fresh roughly chopped cilantro
- 2 cups of chicken broth

Directions:

1. With the burner on high heat, boil the carrots in a saucepan till it is soft. That should take about 3 minutes. Then drain the water out, leaving just the carrots. Add the fish sauce and chick broth to the carrots and stir.

2. Add the turmeric, tomato, coconut cream, celery, curry powder, and coriander to the mix. Boil everything over high heat.

3. Once it has boiled, reduce the heat to low. Cover the pan and while stirring occasionally, allow it to simmer for 20 minutes.

4. Add the cilantro, fish, and ginger to the mix and stir well so that they are covered with the mix.

5. Allow it to cook over medium heat for additional 5 minutes till the fish becomes flaky.

6. Serve hot.

Beef with Spinach and Sweet Potatoes

40 MINUTES 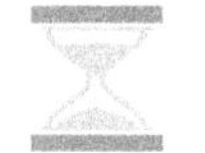

30 MINUTES 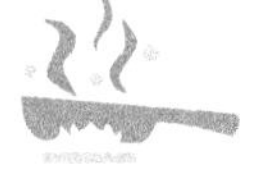

1 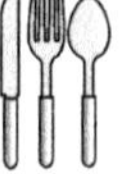

Are you looking for the perfect balance of carbs, high-quality fat, and protein with vegetables? Then this is a dish you would thoroughly enjoy.

Nutritional Information per serving:

Total Carbs: 31.0g; Protein: 43.6g; Fat: 49.4g; Fibre: 5.7g; Sodium: 487mg; Calories:779

Ingredients:

- ¼ tbsp. of chili powder
- ¼ tbsp. of salt
- ¼ tbsp. of freshly ground black pepper
- ½ tbsp. of ground turmeric
- 1/3 cup of toasted pumpkin seeds
- ½ pound of half inch cubes sweet potatoes
- 1 ½ cups of fresh baby spinach
- 2 tbsp. of rice wine vinegar
- 3 tbsp. of olive oil
- 3 tbsp. of pure maple syrup
- 1 pound of organic beef tenderloin

Directions:

1. Cut the beef tenderloin into four medallions, then season it with salt and pepper.

2. Get a cast iron skillet on a burner set to medium heat. Pour two teaspoons of the olive oil and heat it for 1 minute. Transfer the seasoned meat into the skillet and allow to cook on both sides for six minutes till it is medium-rare done. Take out the beef and cover with foil.

3. Using the same skillet, pour the remaining one teaspoon of oil into it and add the sweet potatoes. Set the burner to medium heat and let it cook for 15 minutes. Once the potatoes turn brown, add the turmeric and chili powder. Stir it all together and allow it to cook for one more minute.

4. Add the pure maple syrup and the vinegar to the potatoes and stir. Taking ½ cup of the spinach at a time, add them into the skillet with stirring till you add all the spinach.

5. Cook it for two more minutes, then take off the heat. Pour the spinach and potatoes into plates and add the beef on top of it with the pumpkin seeds.

Flaky Mediterranean Fish with Veggies

Preparation time: 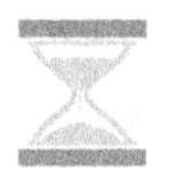	Cooking time: 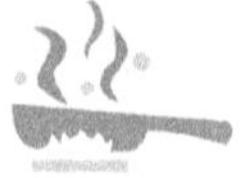	Servings: 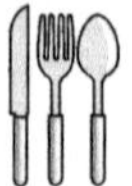
35 MINUTES	12 MINUTES	4

Served with potatoes and salad, this recipe is a meal I personally relish. The flavors are so yummy and tasty. Perfect for dinner after a long day. Tasty and healthy is not an adjective we describe many dishes with, but this? Absolutely!!!

Nutritional Information per serving:

Total Carbs: 5.5g; Protein: 16.5g; Fat: 14.8g; Fibre: 1.8g; Sodium: 533mg; Calories:230

Ingredients:

- ¼ tbsp. of sea salt
- ¼ cup of thinly sliced fresh basil
- ½ tbsp. of freshly ground black pepper
- 1 cup of grated zucchini
- 4 skinless Atlantic cod fillets, 3.5 ounce
- 4 tbsp. of olive oil
- 4 tbsp. of dry white wine
- 4 whole basil leaves
- 10 black sliced olives
- 20 halved cherry tomatoes.

Directions:

1. Preheat the oven to a temperature of 205 degrees Celsius.
2. We need to cut out four heart-shaped parchment paper. Start by cutting a 17 x 11 inches piece of parchment paper with scissors. Fold one side of the long edge to the other side. Then cut out the heart shape from the folded paper, with the center of the fold being the center of the heart as well. Do this till you get four pieced of heart-shaped parchment paper.
3. Set the heart shaped parchment papers on a large cutting board. Along one half of the heart, place the Atlantic cod leaving enough space around the edges. Do this for all four hearts and set aside.
4. Pour the sliced basil, tomatoes, pepper, zucchini, olives, and salt in a medium sized bowl and stir well to mix.
5. Place the spice mix on each of the fish fillets on the hearts. Take the free half of the heart and fold over the fish. Fold and crimp the edges of the hearts tightly together. Be sure to leave a couple of inches unfolded at the sharp end of the heart. Pour in 1 tablespoon of oil and wine through the unfolded edge for each of the hearts. Once you are done, fold and crimp the sharp edge as well, then transfer it into the oven.
6. Allow it to bake for 12 minutes, then check if the fish is cooked through. Do that by poking it with a toothpick; the toothpick would easily slide through. Once it is done, take it out and open the packets carefully.
7. Garnish with the whole basil leaves. Serve hot.

Stuffed Peppers with Ground Turkey

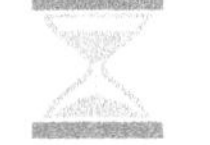

Preparation time:

55 MINUTES

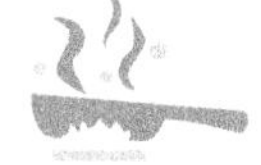

Cooking time:

40 MINUTES

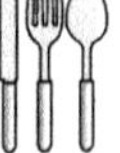

Servings:

1

This is one of those dishes that you prepare and refrigerate in advance. You can choose to add extra vegetables to the recipe.

Nutritional Information per serving:

Total Carbs: 31.0g; Protein: 43.6g; Fat: 49.4g; Fibre: 5.7g; Sodium: 487mg; Calories:779

Ingredients:

- ½ tbsp. of ground cumin
- 1 cup of cooked brown rice
- 1 pound of ground turkey
- 1 tbsp. of smoked paprika
- 1 tbsp. of olive oil
- 1 tbsp. of garlic-infused oil
- 1 ½ tbsp. of chili powder
- 2 tbsp. of pine nuts
- 2 tbsp. of melted coconut oil
- 2 chopped medium sized Roma tomatoes
- 3 tbsp. of sugar-free salsa
- 3 tbsp. of fresh chopped cilantro
- 3 large stemmed, seeded and halved bell peppers (yellow, green, and orange)
- 6 slices of goat cheese

Directions:

1. Preheat the oven to a temperature of 190 degrees Celsius.

2. Get a skillet on a burner set to medium heat. Pour the olive oil in it and heat for a minute. Put the turkey and cook for about 7 minutes till it is brown.

3. Add the tomatoes, pine nuts, and half of the garlic oil to the skillet and cook for 3 minutes.

4. While stirring, add the brown rice, paprika, cumin, cilantro, garlic oil, and chili powder to the skillet. Then turn off the heat.

5. Scoop the rice mixture into the halved bell peppers and brush the peppers with coconut oil. Put them on a baking dish and put the slice of goat cheese on top. Cover the baking dish loosely with foil.

6. Bake the peppers for 40 minutes toil they are tender. Remove the pepper from the oven, garnish with salsa and serve.

Salmon with Herbs

Preparation time:		Cooking time:		Servings:	
35 MINUTES		25 MINUTES	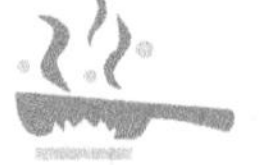	1	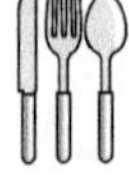

The choice of salmon in this dish is because of the plenty omega-3 fatty acids it contains. Based on your preference, though, you can choose any fish for this recipe.

Nutritional Information per serving:

Total Carbs: 1.5g; Protein: 22.8g; Fat: 26.2g; Fibre: 0.5g; Sodium: 197mg; Calories:342

Ingredients:

- ¼ cup of fresh flat-leaf parsley
- ¼ tbsp. of salt
- ¼ cup of fresh chopped dill
- ¼ cup plus two tablespoons of olive oil
- ½ tbsp. of freshly ground black pepper
- 1 pound of salmon fillet
- 2 tbsp. of fresh thyme leaves
- 2 tbsp. of roughly chopped fresh rosemary
- 2 tbsp. of freshly squeezed lemon juice

Directions:

1. Preheat the oven to a temperature of 120 degrees Celsius.
2. Lay the salmon with the skin side on a greased baking sheet and sprinkle with salt and pepper.
3. Get a food processor. Pour in the rosemary, thyme, parsley, dill, olive oil, and lemon juice and pulse for about 15 seconds. Scoop the paste from the processor and spread it on the salmon.
4. Based on the thickness of the salmon, bake it for 22-28 minutes. Check for the flakiness of the fish. If the thickest part flakes easily, the salmon is done.
5. Lift the fish gently off the baking dish with a spatula and set it down on a cutting board. Cut the fish into equal pieces and serve.

Chicken Burgers

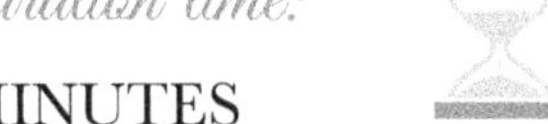

Preparation time:
15 MINUTES

Cooking time:
10 MINUTES

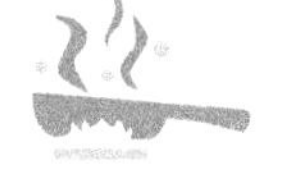

Servings:
1

We all know and love burgers. They are easy to make and store and can be made readily available when we need them. You can also add a spin to it by selecting your own choice of spices and meat.

Nutritional Information per serving:

Total Carbs: 1.2g; Protein: 21.9g; Fat: 13.9g; Fibre: 0.9g; Sodium: 480mg; Calories:224

Ingredients:

- ¼ cup of grated parmesan cheese
- ½ tbsp. of salt
- ½ tbsp. ground white pepper
- 1 tbsp. of olive oil
- 1 large, whisked egg
- 1 pound of ground chicken

Directions:

1. Get a big bowl and pour in all the ingredients leaving out the oil. Mix it together with your hands till it is well combined.

2. Shape the mixture with your hands into four patties.

3. Heat the olive oil in a large skillet for one minute before adding the patties. Cook both sides for 5 minutes each till they are well browned.

4. Serve hot.

Spinach and Feta-Stuffed Chicken Breasts

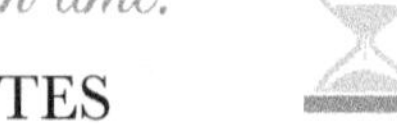

Preparation time:

35 MINUTES

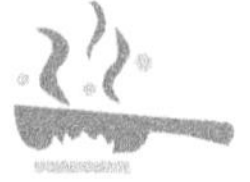

Cooking time:

30 MINUTES

Servings:

2

With just 30 minutes, you get to prepare a delicious dinner with just a few ingredients. It is so easy to make.

Nutritional Information per serving:

Total Carbs: 5.2g; Protein: 35.8g; Fat: 24.1g; Fibre: 1.8g; Sodium: 423mg; Calories:395

Ingredients:

- ½ cup of crumbled feta cheese
- 1 cup of almond meal
- 1 cup of fresh spinach leaves
- 1 large egg
- 1 tbsp. of garlic-infused olive oil
- 2 skinless chicken breasts, boneless.

Directions:

1. Preheat the oven to a temperature of 180 degrees Celsius.

2. With a skillet over low heat, heat the olive oil for a minute. Then add the spinach and allow to cook for about 3 minutes until it is soft. Add the feta cheese to the skillet and stir before you remove it from the heat.

3. Pound each boneless chicken breast to about a quarter of an inch. Scoop the spinach mix from the skillet into each chicken breast. Fold the chicken breast around the mix and hold it in place with a toothpick.

4. Break the egg into a bowl and beat lightly. Set it aside.

5. Add the almond meal into a separate bowl. Take a chicken breast and roll carefully in the egg till it is well covered. Tap off the excess egg, then roll the same chicken breast in the almond meat till it is totally coated as well. Place the covered chicken on a casserole dish. Do the same for the other chicken breast.

6. Bake the chicken breasts for 30 minutes and serve hot.

Slow cooker Chicken Tagine

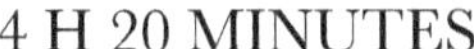

Preparation time: 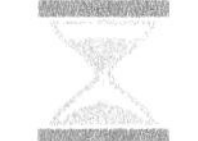
4 H 20 MINUTES

Cooking time: 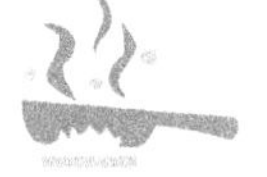
4 H 5 MINUTES

Servings: 
2

This traditional dish is popular in Morocco and some other places in North Africa. The recipe is easy to prepare and a joy to consume.

Nutritional Information per serving:

Total Carbs: 21.5g; Protein: 34.2g; Fat: 15.8g; Fibre: 3.8g; Sodium: 810mg; Calories:381

Ingredients:

- 1/8 tbsp. of asafetida powder, wheat free
- ¼ tbsp. of sea salt
- ¼ tbsp. of freshly ground black pepper
- 1/3 cup of rinsed and thoroughly drained canned chickpeas
- 1 tbsp. of olive oil
- 1 tbsp. of ground cinnamon
- 1 drained 14-ounce can of whole tomatoes
- 1 lemon that has been sliced into wedges
- 1 quart of chicken stock
- 1 tbsp. of fresh chopped flat-leaf parsley
- 1 ½ tbsp. of ground turmeric
- 1 ½ tbsp. of saffron
- 1 ½ tbsp. of sweet paprika
- 1 ½ tbsp. of ground ginger
- 1 ½ tbsp. of ground allspice
- 1 ½ tbsp. of ground coriander
- 2 tbsp. of ground cardamom
- 4 skinless 5-ounce size boneless chicken thighs cut in half.

Directions:

1. Set the burner to medium heat. Place a skillet over it and add the turmeric, paprika, cinnamon, allspice, cardamom, and coriander. Toast them all in the skillet till the flavor starts to come out. This would take you about 2 minutes. Stir them well, remove the heat, and set them aside.

2. Once the toasted spice mix has cooled down, sprinkle it with the salt, pepper, and asafetida on the halved chicken thighs. Make sure you sprinkle on both sides of the chicken thighs.

3. Heat oil in a large skillet for a minute on medium heat, then add the chicken thighs to it. Sear each side until it turns brown, then remove from the skillet and place in a 4 to 6-quart slow cooker.

4. Toast the ginger for 2 minutes in the small skillet on medium heat, then add to the slow cooker as well.

5. Finally, add the other ingredients to the slow cooker – the chicken stock, the tomatoes, saffron, and chickpeas. Cook everything on high heat for four hours.

6. Remove the heat and serve. Add the parsley and lemon to garnish.

Lemon Thyme Chicken

Preparation time: 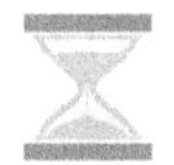
50 MINUTES

Cooking time: 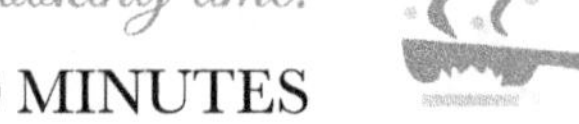
40 MINUTES

Servings: 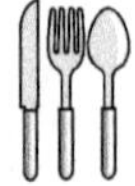
4

Thyme is known to reduce the cholesterol levels in the body and reduce our blood pressure too. It is even known to improve the mood sometimes. We have paired this awesome herb with lemons to give you a delicious tasting citrus chicken dish.

Nutritional Information per serving:

Total Carbs: 2.3g; Protein: 58.6g; Fat: 22.5g; Fibre: 0.5g; Sodium: 280mg; Calories:480

Ingredients:

- ¼ tbsp. of sea salt
- ½ tbsp. of freshly ground black pepper
- 1 tbsp. of melted and unsalted organic butter
- 2 tbsp. of fresh thyme leaves
- 3 medium sized lemons cut in half
- 4 chicken thighs with skin
- 4 chicken drumsticks with skin
- 6 torn fresh basil leaves
- Zest of 1 medium sized lemon

Directions:

1. Preheat the oven to a temperature of 190 degrees Celsius.

2. Place the chicken in a bowl. Add salt, pepper, lemon zest, butter, and squeeze the juice from the halved lemons. Toss it all together; make sure to use your hands so that everything seeps into the chicken, then place the chicken on a baking dish.

3. Bake for forty minutes, making sure to baste the chicken every 10-minute interval till the skin is crisp and the meat cooked.

4. Remove from the oven and garnish with the basil leaves before serving.